Black Health

BIOETHICS FOR SOCIAL JUSTICE

Quill Kukla, Georgetown University and
Sean A. Valles, Michigan State University

Published in the Series

Black Health
The Social, Political, and Cultural Determinants of Black People's Health
Keisha Ray

Black Health

The Social, Political, and Cultural Determinants of Black People's Health

KEISHA RAY

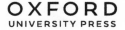

OXFORD
UNIVERSITY PRESS

OXFORD
UNIVERSITY PRESS

Oxford University Press is a department of the University of Oxford. It furthers
the University's objective of excellence in research, scholarship, and education
by publishing worldwide. Oxford is a registered trade mark of Oxford University
Press in the UK and certain other countries.

Published in the United States of America by Oxford University Press
198 Madison Avenue, New York, NY 10016, United States of America.

© Oxford University Press 2023

CIP data is on file at the Library of Congress

ISBN 978-0-19-762027-4 (pbk.)
ISBN 978-0-19-762026-7 (hbk.)

DOI: 10.1093/oso/9780197620267.001.0001

Contents

Contents

Series Foreword

Bioethics has, in recent years, become radically more world-responsive in its scope and mission. It has become intertwined with other disciplines and subfields such as political philosophy, environmental ethics, critical race theory, philosophy of science, gender theory, disability studies, and public health. It has added many new lenses to its toolkit and dramatically increased its attention to power relationships, systematic and structural oppressions, and the material and social conditions of existence.

The changing scope and texture of bioethics is in part a response to a changing world. We are increasingly aware that "health" is much broader than in-clinic health care. The model of the doctor as a benign authority and privileged source of information that undergirded much early bioethics has given way to a much messier story about multiple sources of information, conflicting authority, capitalism, and power, in which doctors play a smaller and more vexed role. Our health is determined less than once thought by the quality of one's healthcare, and more than once thought by social position, the material environment including pollutants, food access, transportation options, stress, and stigmas. Inclusive models of health have been urging that health encompasses much more than freedom from disease: sexual pleasure, social connectedness, food security, safety on the street, and more. Thus, bioethics must broaden its view well beyond the confines of the clinic, to encompass large scale social structures and material and economic pressures. This makes it inevitable that high-quality bioethics will be intertwined with environmental ethics, political philosophy, public health, urban studies, and more.

We live in an increasingly cosmopolitan, connected world. Accordingly, society is increasingly sensitive to demographic differences and how they impact health and experience. Bioethics has slowly but surely adopted a more global and intersectional perspective that has revealed new ethical issues surrounding health and deepened old ones. For example, bioethicists are increasingly alert to the cultural imperialism that governs much international research, and sensitive to concerns about climate justice on a global scale. Ethical issues that cross international boundaries and huge power and resource divides such as sex trafficking, international surrogacy and adoption, and medical tourism are receiving increasing attention. Meanwhile, we are becoming better at attending to the intersectional influence of race, disability, sexual orientation, body shape, gender identity, and other social positions and embodied identities on health, values, and experience. This new global and intersectional focus goes in two directions: On the one hand, it shows that many of our intuitions and solutions that may "feel" universal can't be generalized across perspectives, situations, and regions. On the other, there are critical ethical problems that simply don't emerge as visible until we broaden our vision in these ways, such as the exploitation of the bodily labor of citizens of poor countries to benefit the health of those from rich countries, or how trade laws or climate policies may worsen global inequity and health harms to low-resource areas.

Our driving vision for this book series is to show the deep and inextricable links between bioethical issues and larger social patterns, including structural oppression and power relationships, inequities in everyday life, and the complexities of identity. Our belief is that a social justice lens reveals new bioethical issues and deepens and illuminates old ones. We take this series to be doing active work to redefine and give new and updated unity to bioethics as a field, reframing public engagement and social justice as central to the field, rather than marginal concerns.

Series Editors

Quill Kukla, PhD, MA, Professor of Philosophy and Disability Studies and Senior Research Scholar in the Kennedy Institute of Ethics, Georgetown University

Sean A. Valles, PhD, Director and Associate Professor, Center for Bioethics and Social Justice, College of Human Medicine, Michigan State University

Series Editorial Board

Rosemarie Garland-Thomson, PhD, Professor Emerita of English and Bioethics, Emory University

Anita Ho, PhD, MPH, Associate Professor of Population and Public Health, University of British Columbia

Serene Khader, PhD, Jay Newman Chair in Philosophy of Culture and Associate Professor of Philosophy, City University of New York

Jonathan Michael Kaplan, PhD, Professor of Philosophy, Oregon State University

Joan McGregor, PhD, Professor of Historical, Philosophical, and Religious Studies, and Professor in the Julie Ann Wrigley Global Institute of Sustainability, Arizona State University

Andrea Pitts, PhD, Associate Professor of Philosophy and Affiliated Associate Professor of Africana Studies, Latin American Studies, and Women's and Gender Studies, University of North Carolina at Charlotte

Kyle Powys Whyte, PhD, Professor of Environment and Sustainability and George Willis Pack Professor at the University of Michigan School for Environment and Sustainability

Preface

I started teaching bioethics fifteen years ago. As a graduate student instructor, I had a lot to learn about developing a curriculum, but I knew that I wanted to teach about racial disparities in health outcomes. I knew that I had my own experiences with medical racism, my family and friends told me about racist physicians they encountered while trying to get care, and countless stories on social media and online news sources told of poor health connected to institutional racism in health care. I knew it was important and I wanted my students to know about it too, but I did not know where to begin to start developing this part of my syllabus.

I tried to find easy-to-read, short, scholarly, and undergraduate-friendly articles that would be appropriate for my students. I hoped to find one text that provided the information and stories that I had been reading on the internet about Black, Latinx, and Indigenous people's interactions with health care, but I could not find it. It was even difficult to find multiple sources that I could piece together. Instead, I had to take my own knowledge and information from articles and books too difficult for undergraduates, and create presentations for my students. But I never felt this was enough. Students always wanted to know more. They wanted to read about racial disparities in health and not just sit through my best attempt to present them with the historical facts and the contemporary issues.

Additionally, my bioethics colleagues would often tell me that although they did not have expertise in racial disparities in health, particularly those affecting Black people, they realized the need to teach these topics in their classes. But they did not feel that they could do the topic justice and wished that they had a book that could do the heavy-lifting for them.

As I started researching and publishing articles about Black health I would get requests from people in my life for books that they could read about Black people's health, but were also easy to read. Many of these requests came from Black people who wanted to know more about the history of their people's relationship with health care. Additionally, when I would give presentations about Black health, attendees would say they wished other people in their families could hear or watch my presentations.

Black Health was born out of these experiences; it was born from a need for an easy-to-read, narrative-informed text about the social determinants of Black people's health that is accessible to people from all walks of life. Public scholarship is at the heart of all my academic work, and *Black Health* is an extension of my commitment to making my work accessible to as many people as possible. The story of Black health is meant for everyone and should not be hidden in the ivory tower of academia. Rather the violence health care systems and public health institutions have displayed in the past and continue to impose on Black individuals and Black communities must be shared with the public.

For too long, bioethics has ignored this violence and abuse and instead has chosen to focus on a few historical instances such as the Tuskegee Syphilis Study and the story of Henrietta Lacks. Although both are examples of inhumane treatment of Black people whose effects are still felt in Black people's relationship with health care, medicine, and science, it is the stories of disregard, violence, disrespect, and abuse that we hear from our families, friends, colleagues, or those of our own experiences that perpetuate the poor relationship between Black people and health care. It is these experiences that continue to hurt our access to health and happiness. I wish to set bioethics anew in *Black Health*— to tell our stories and make it so that they are a standard practice in bioethics and not something we ignore and sweep under the rug. I wish to allow Black people to tell their own stories, rather than have someone else give a watered-downed retelling of our experiences. I wish to see Black people's experiences of poor health in all of its heartache and pain and force bioethics to reckon with our truths, and more importantly the truths of health care and public health, namely that they have killed, mutilated, and violated Black people and forced us to keep quiet. But not anymore. *Black Health* is a reckoning for bioethics. *Black Health* is Black Bioethics.

Introduction

What Is Black Health?

Of all the forms of inequality, injustice in health care is the
most shocking and inhuman because it often results in
physical death.

　　　　　　　　　　　　　　　　—Martin Luther King, Jr.

*Jason Hargrove, a Black man and bus driver in Detroit, Michigan,
died of COVID-19 on April 1, 2020. Four days before his death a self-
recorded video of himself went viral on the internet. In it Hargrove
complained about a rider on his bus who he felt was not taking
COVID-19 seriously as he witnessed her freely coughing. Just a few
weeks before Hargrove's death, Detroit bus drivers went on strike because they did not have enough protective equipment like face masks.
They voiced just how imperative this equipment was to performing
their job, while at the same time protecting their health since they
often transport[1] sick people to hospitals and see sick people even before doctors see them.*

Hargrove joins the 14 percent of Black Americans who are a part
of the over million total American deaths from COVID-19 (as
of May 2022).[2] Since March 11, 2020, when the World Health
Organization (WHO) declared the spread of COVID-19, a novel
coronavirus, a pandemic,[3] preliminary research shows that Black
people (along with some other racial minority groups) have had
disproportionate rates of infection, hospitalization, and deaths
from COVID-19 compared to their total population size.[4] As the

Black Health. Keisha Ray, Oxford University Press. © Oxford University Press 2023.
DOI: 10.1093/oso/9780197620267.003.0001

pandemic continues, it is suspected that Black people will continue to die from the disease at a higher rate than White people when we adjust for factors like age.

Why do American Black people generally have worse health than American White people? To answer this question, first, anyone interested in health justice must abandon any notion that Black people have inferior bodies or minds that are inherently susceptible to disease and illness because they are Black. This is simply false racial science that has been used to abuse and mistreat Black people since our African ancestors were brought to America on slave ships and White settlers needed a reason to justify their inhumane actions. A genuine investigation into the status of Black people's health requires us to acknowledge that *race* has always been a powerful social category. Race largely predetermines individuals' social and political power and access to resources needed for health and wellbeing. And as a group, Black people have been intentionally denied this power and access. For example, the Centers for Disease Control and Prevention (CDC) cite differing social and economic conditions between Black and White people as the reason for the disproportionate number of deaths of Black people with COVID-19. These differing conditions include a lack of access to testing and care; higher rates of comorbidities such as hypertension, diabetes, and obesity (all of which can have social origins); lesser disposable income; and poorer living conditions. Black people are also more likely than White people to work jobs that are considered essential to our daily living such as grocery store workers and janitorial workers. These essential jobs give them more contact with people and a higher likelihood of exposure to COVID-19, yet they are less likely to have jobs with paid sick time.[5] When people do not have paid sick time, they may continue to work despite being sick because they need the income, but at the same time possibly infect coworkers and customers. These social and economic differences between Black and White Americans existed long before the COVID-19 pandemic; however, the pandemic created an opportunity for these inequities to create new unjust differences in health. These unjust differences in health are often referred to as health disparities, which the American Medical Association (AMA) defines as "a higher burden of illness, injury, disability or mortality experienced by one group relative to another."[6] In this particular instance, COVID-19 created racial disparities in health between White and Black people, with Black people on the losing end, but it also worsened pre-existing racial disparities in health between the two groups.

Historically, for many individuals, being Black has not conferred social power or access to adequate social resources necessary for health. In fact, laws have been enacted and customs have been implemented to actively withhold social power and resources from Black people. For example, laws and practices like redlining and gerrymandering have been used to keep Black people out of White and wealthy neighborhoods as well as keep Black children from attending wealthier schools. Historical and contemporary laws that make it difficult or impossible for Black people to vote in democratic elections continue to take political power away from Black individuals and communities.[7] Systemic racism, oppression, and White supremacy in American institutions have largely been the perpetrators of differing social power and access to resources between Black people and White people. It is these systemic inequities that created the conditions needed for poor health outcomes for Black people to persist.[5] An examination of social inequities like these reveals that it is no accident that Black people have poorer health than White people; instead in America, almost every institution has been designed to withhold what Black people need for proper health and wellbeing.

Scholars have produced an abundance of data on the status of Black people's health in the United States.[8] One of the most notable pieces of research on the topic came in 1985 in the Report of the Secretary's Task Force on Black People and Minority Health, aka the Heckler Report. It is largely responsible for bringing the issue of inequities in Black people's health to the forefront of ethical discussions. The Heckler report noted Black people's unequal experiences of adverse health, delivery of health care, and health care outcomes.[9] Additional data accumulated since the Heckler Report clearly demonstrates that Black people's health outcomes, life expectancy, and experiences with health care are inequitable to that of most White people's health outcomes and experiences with health care. These unjust differences in health outcomes, including the prevalence of comorbidities and mortality and differences in access to health care, are what scholars refer to as racial disparities in health. Typically, discussions of racial disparities in health compare the health of people of color to that of White people as White people generally have better health outcomes and receive better health care than other racial groups. Although this book is about Black people's health, I sometimes compare Black people's health to White people's health to (1) demonstrate the stark disparities between the two groups of people, and (2) demonstrate that health care systems, laws, and policies can work for people, they just do not work for Black people and that it is not by accident, but by design. But this by no means should be viewed as White people being the standard we should all use for Black people's health goals. Instead, we should want better for everyone, but right now people interested in advocating for health equity, need to strive for equity for Black people.

The overall goal of this text is to provide a succinct discussion of the social causes of Black people's generally poor health outcomes and their lesser access to health care. There is, however, a point of view—Black people's multiple identities (race, class, and gender)—that intersect with anti-Black racism in social institutions to shape their experiences of poor health outcomes. Given this, a singular framework that examines Black health, or Black people's health from the perspective of medical racism or the American law alone, for instance, would ignore the complexity of the problem. In this text I use an intersectional framework[10] that situates Black people's marginalized identities within the social and cultural institutions and practices that shape health. Housing (i.e., the effects of legal and illegal segregation), health care (i.e., health care policies), economics (i.e., the effects of income inequity), and the law (i.e., legal protections for pollutant emitting facilities) are primarily the institutions that shape health and thus are the primary focus of this text. In addition to examining the influence of these institutions, I also examine how other social, political, and cultural forces influence Black people's health outcomes.

To illustrate the intersectional approach of this book and keep Black people's experiences at the forefront, each chapter includes stories and testimonies from and/or about Black people. These stories offer firsthand accounts of how Black people's identities influence their health outcomes and experiences with health care. They also reveal the human toll of disparate health outcomes. Readers will get to read their stories of how poor health limits their wellbeing, their propensity for social mobility, and the ability to take advantage of life's opportunities. In short, this approach humanizes the examination of Black health during a time when so often Black people's humanity is denied.

This introduction chapter sets the stage for the core chapters. It provides the necessary background to take part in the discussions held in each of the core chapters. Although each chapter can be read without first reading this chapter or any of the others, I would recommend reading this chapter before embarking on the others. In the following sections of this chapter, I discuss the origins of race and racial disparities in health and the social determinants of health, and provide summaries of each core chapter.

Race and Racism in Medicine

Almost all biologists, anthropologists, race scholars, and other types of scholars now agree that race as a biological category of humans has been scientifically disproven. Instead, most scholars now believe race to be a social construct.[11] This means that race, at least when referring to humans, does not match onto biologically distinct human groupings. In other words, nature did not bestow certain unique traits onto humans that can then be grouped together based on these natural traits. This is not to say that genetic differences do not exist; genetic differences do exist. It's just that our genetic differences do not perfectly map onto race as we use it today; it is not a product of evolutionary biology, nor supported by science (as applied to humans). Instead, race is an idea created by humans for human purposes and one of those human purposes was slavery.

Some scholars believe that a biological explanation of race was created to justify enslaving Africans.[12] In the eighteenth century when the concept of race was beginning to be applied to humans to group biologically distinct people, race became an important economic tool for economic exploitation.[13] To further support and legitimize the economic benefits that enslaved Africans brought to slave owners, particularly in the American south, the concept of race as a biologically real construct, that is, an entity found in science, was eventually advanced in the general public and eventually supported by physicians in their writings and medical practices as well as reinforced by some theological doctrines.[14]

During America's enslavement of Africans (and subsequent African Americans), physicians had an intimate relationship with slavery. In fact, slavery made physicians very wealthy. They used their racially motivated medical theories and diagnoses to support the justification of slavery and to care for slaves so that they could continue to turn a profit for White slave owners. And in return White slave owners made physicians very wealthy.[15] This relationship between physicians and slavery was built on physicians preaching about biological differences between Africans and African Americans (i.e., Black people) and White Americans. For instance, physicians believed that Black people had feeble minds making them susceptible to some mental disorders like schizophrenia, but not susceptible to what were considered high-functioning mental disorders like depression.[16] When it came to their beliefs about Black bodies, on the one hand they believed Black bodies were feeble and thus more susceptible to disease and illness than White people. But on the other hand, they believed that their bodies were strong and sturdy, making them especially able to endure difficult labor on slave plantations and punishments like whippings. These beliefs culminated in the reigning belief at the time that Black people's inferior biology made them suitable to be slaves for the more intellectually superior White people.[17] Without physicians advocating for Black people's inferiority, slavery likely would not have been a mainstay in America for as long as it was. American physicians were instrumental in maintaining and cultivating Black people's enslavement and false beliefs about Black people's humanity. This intimate relationship between medicine and slavery set the stage for medicine's relationship with Black people but also for the law's relationship with Black people.

Different laws and policies were enacted to support the belief in Black inferiority and as such to keep Black people separate from White people. One such law was the "one drop rule." The one drop rule, enacted in 1662, was the policy that one drop of "Black blood" makes a person Black. Another way of saying this is that any person who had an ancestor of African origin, no matter how distant, was considered a Black person for any legal or social purposes such as Census reporting.[18] Although it was declared unconstitutional in 1967,[19] in 1985 the one drop rule was used to declare a woman legally Black. In the case of *Jane Doe vs. Louisiana*, Susie Guillory Phipps was denied a passport because she declared on her application that she was White when her birth certificate said she was Colored, that is, Black. She asked the state of Louisiana to change her deceased parents' birth certificates to indicate that they were White so that she could change her race to White. She argued that she lived as a White woman and should be able to change the designation on her birth certificate. The courts denied Phipps' request based on the information that in 1770 a White French planter named Jean Gregoire Guillory used his social position of power to force his wife's enslaved African woman, Margarita, to be his mistress. Since Margarita, a Black woman, was Susie Guillory Phipps' great-great-great-great grandmother, Louisiana courts considered Phipps to be a Black woman.[20]

Laws like the "one drop rule" or laws that prohibited marriages between Black and White people were meant to keep the White gene pool pure. These laws were meant to keep Black people, including people of bi-racial ancestry from identifying as White people, thus being entitled to the legal and social benefits (e.g., inheritance, visibility, social power) of being White in America. Specific references to the one drop rule may have lost steam in our culture, but the basic idea is still rampant in our American culture. The one-drop rule can still be seen in the ways we classify and view people of bi-racial ancestry based on their skin color (e.g., Barack Obama is publicly viewed as a Black man even though he is of bi-racial ancestry), or the ways legal documents often force people to identify as one race.

Medicine and biomedical research still occasionally use the concept of race to categorize people based on genetic differences among the human population,[21] although with less (but still some) White supremacist undertones. The idea behind some biomedical research is that the genes that determine race can also tell us what diseases a person is susceptible to and even shed light on how to treat people for diseases. Although our genetic make-up can determine how likely we are to develop certain genetic disorders, our race does not determine our susceptibility to genetic disorders. Furthermore, racial categories like White, Black, or Hispanic do not denote unique genetic variation. For instance, there can be more genetic variation between two Black people than between a White and Black person. Genetically speaking, we are all more alike than different. Regardless of race and geographic origin, all humans share 99.9 percent of known genetic factors. There are patterns in genetic characteristics, but our current racial categories do not map onto these genetic patterns.[22]

People who want to ignore scientific research dispelling the biological explanations of race may try to use sickle cell anemia as an example of a biological basis for race. Sickle cell anemia is a very painful red blood cell disorder that affects 20 million people in the world and about a hundred thousand Americans. People with the disease have atypical shaped red blood cells, which causes symptoms like anemia, shortness of breath, and even death. Most people who have sickle cell anemia have African ancestry (but it is also fairly common in people of Hispanic and Mediterranean origin).[23] Sickle cell anemia, however, only accounts for 0.3 percent of deaths in the Black population. Furthermore, scholars believe that even though this disease is more common in Black people than White people, sickle cell anemia's prevalence in people of sub-Saharan African ancestry, in part, is because of the interaction between inherited factors and social environment. Sickle cell anemia seems to have developed as protection against environmental conditions evidenced by higher rates of sickle cell anemia occurring in people who have origins in places with high rates of malaria.[24] If anything, sickle cell anemia's higher rates in the Black population is evidence of the impact our social environment can have on our health and not on the biological existence of race.

Because most scholars have abandoned a biological explanation of race for a social explanation of race, in this book I will also use a social understanding of race; however, just because race is a social construct does not mean it does not matter in our lives. When discussing Black health, and really any other topic that concerns race, it is important to refrain from dismissing race as irrelevant simply because it is a social construct. Like other social constructs such as money and clothing, or ideals such as fairness and justice, social constructs still have power and influence over our daily lives. Therefore, labeling an entity or ideal as a "social construct" does not mean we should ignore it. In fact, ignoring a social construct like race leaves room for ignorant views about people of color to persist and no way to discuss how these views affect the lives of specific populations of humans. Therefore, in this text I rely on an understanding that race is a complex, always evolving, and socially constructed idea that we have created to group people together based on a shared history, culture, language, and sometimes a range of skin colors (among other things) for social and political purposes. Although race is a loaded term, often fraught with value claims, complexities, and a lack of clarity, it is necessary when discussing health disparities that often fall along racial lines. To understand who is most affected and how to help, we have to talk about the role race and racism play in health disparities. So for the purpose of this book, I will use the term race and all of the racial categories that it denotes, like White, Black, Latinx, and Indigenous, while acknowledging its social roots.[25]

Like many other scholars I also rely on a social explanation of race to avoid potential negative social implications associated with biological understandings of race. Biological explanations of race can be harmful to individual people of color, populations of people of color, as well as to the practice and study of biology and medicine. For example, because some form of a biological understanding of race still lingers in medicine, clinicians often rely on a patient's race to diagnose and treat their disease, which can lead to misdiagnoses and improper treatments. I experienced this when I received my diagnosis of hypertension:[26]

> When I was a senior in college I discovered I had hypertension. I went to see a doctor at a family medicine facility and was prescribed a common hypertension drug. While meeting with the doctor in their office, she was very reassuring and told me not to worry that this drug has been known to work very well for Black people.
>
> But this drug did not work for me at all. Consistently my blood pressure readings were 140/120 (what is considered "normal"

varies, but typically 120/80 is the standard). So after taking the drug for a month as instructed, I went back to see my doctor. In that office I encountered an utterly dumbfounded doctor. She just could not believe that the drug did not work for me. She kept saying "I just don't understand. This drug is supposed to work for Black people." She even said "Plus it's cheap, so it's good for poor Black people" without ever asking me about my financial status. My doctor then said that she was going to come up with a new game plan and I was optimistic that something was going to be done about my hypertension. Little did I know that the doctor's "new" game plan was actually the same game plan. Her recommendation: "Let's keep trying because this drug is supposed to work for Black people."

In this encounter my doctor did not see me as an individual person with my own health care needs; before being seen as a person, I was seen as a Black person. Because medicine still relies on the idea that some drugs work better for Black people than other drugs, my doctor was unwilling to explore other care options when her initial care plan did not work for me.

My experience is one example of how a biological explanation of race can prove to be harmful to Black patients and encourage racism in medicine. A social understanding of race, however, does not avoid racism, but it does help us evaluate the concept in a way that makes the problem a matter of how we think about people rather than how nature made people. Each chapter will give a deeper understanding of racism and racial bias, or the negative thoughts and attitudes we have about people, in the context of Black health, but in general, in this book I rely on three widely used definitions of different kinds of racism:

Interpersonal racism refers to the prejudices based on race we apply to people in our daily lives.[27] For example, when racial slurs are used to refer to racialized minorities like Black, Latinx, or Indigenous people.

Institutional racism refers to systems of power that disadvantage racialized minorities by unfairly withholding social goods from them like education, housing, and jobs because of their race, while advantaging White people and unfairly making it easier for them to access social goods because of their race. With this definition, individuals do not have to be racist for institutions to be racist.

Structural racism refers to all of the ways our society encourages racism, particularly in social institutions like housing, education, income, employment, health care, and criminal justice, thereby reinforcing discriminatory behavior and attitudes towards racial groups.[28] Structural racism leads to systemic discrimination that then leads to systemic inequitable access to resources and opportunities based on people's race. Structural racism is therefore the totality of all the effects of different types of racism compounded, leading to negative effects on people's lives.[29]

Scholars tend to focus a lot of attention on *institutional racism* because it can be the hardest to reveal, especially to people who are resistant to acknowledging its existence, as well as the hardest to end. But it also has the most systemic impact on people's lives. In this text, though, I will frequently discuss all three. In particular I discuss how racial biases can turn into interpersonal racism and can affect Black people's mental and physical wellbeing. Institutional racism can also affect people's health by affecting their access to the resources they need for proper health outcomes like access to health care. Both types of racism contribute to structural racism and can affect Black people's long-term health making them all important to discussing the components of Black health.

The ways in which race, class, and gender situate Black people within social institutions and the ways in which institutions confer or withhold social power are all relevant to discussing Black health; but we must begin with a social understanding of race. Because there is no biological basis for race in the human species, we can dispel the belief that there is a biological basis for racial disparities in health and the idea that Black people are unhealthy because of their inherent nature. It is also much easier to rid ourselves of the effects of racism in medicine with policy implementation, education, and training if we treat race as just a way to group people based on shared experiences, culture, history, and so on rather than as a group of people with the same biology, which should then be used as a primary diagnostic and therapeutic tool. This way of thinking about race and racism gives us the space to understand and examine Black health and enforce measures meant to better Black people's overall health and wellbeing.

Disparities and Social Determinants of Health

Health is multifaceted. Health can contribute to wellbeing, making it something that most people desire. But health is more than just how our bodies and minds function. Where we live, with whom we live, and how we live can all have an impact on our health. Our social lives can either encourage illness and disease or encourage health and wellbeing. How healthy we are and how much wellbeing we have are directly related to influences on our lives that go beyond our biology.

The social component of health, or social determinants of health, are the social, political, and economic goods, behaviors, and resources that help shape our health. The World Health Organization defines them as "the conditions in which people are born, grow, live, work and age. These circumstances are shaped by the distribution of money, power and resources at global, national and local levels."[30] Table I.1 lists, in no particular order, common social determinants of health that can generally be divided into four categories: education and employment, housing and environment,

Table I.1. Social Determinants of Health

1. Education/Literacy	8. Income
2. Employment	9. No racism/discrimination
3. Housing/Neighborhood safety	10. No close proximity to polluted areas
4. Transportation	11. Clean air and water
5. Recreation	12. Technology
6. Childhood experiences	13. Social order
7. Social relationships/Support	14. Medical care

Source: Public Health Agency of Canada, "Social Determinants of Health and Health Inequalities," Government of Canada, October 7, 2020, https://www.canada.ca/en/public-health/services/health-promotion/population-health/what-determines-health.html; Office of Disease Prevention and Health Promotion, "Social Determinants of Health," HealthyPeople.gov, 2014, https://www.healthypeople.gov/2020/topics-objectives/topic/social-determinants-of-health.

behaviors, and social goods. The general idea is that access to these social determinants can contribute to health and encourage, or at least not hinder, our overall mental and physical health and wellbeing. However, when we do not have access to the social determinants of health, our health and wellbeing suffer.

The social determinants of health are necessary for proper health, but they often intertwine. For example, access to quality education can lead to access to adequate employment, which can help people have an adequate income that gives us the finances to secure safe housing for ourselves and our families. Furthermore, if we live in safe neighborhoods, we are more likely to have access to public transportation; clean, unpolluted air and water; and safe recreation areas, such as parks and playgrounds. In their absence, however, the social determinants of health can lead to poor health like when negative childhood experiences or childhood trauma increases adults' risk for cardiovascular disease and premature mortality.[31] The social determinants of health often work together to either support or not support our health, but all are essential to healthy, happy living.

Although all of the social determinants of health are important, racism deserves extra consideration. To unpack this a little further, a person's race is often a predictor of their access to other social determinants of health. For instance, because of social and political inequities created by racist policies and poor social arrangement, Black people are more likely than White people to work low-paying jobs that do not provide health insurance, which lessens their access to medical care.[32] Black people, regardless of income, are also more likely to live in poorer neighborhoods that have disproportionate rates of violence, more air and noise pollution, and less access to recreation areas.[33] Although for White people more income typically means more access to good health, for Black people this is rarely true. For example, when researchers adjust for socioeconomic status, Black people still have poorer health than White people.[34] This means that for Black people, more income does not always mean better health.

Racism is also a social determinant of health, particularly for people of color like Black, Latinx, Asian, and Indigenous people because it is a predictor for their experiences with the negative health effects of racism and other forms of discrimination. For Black people, in particular, experiences with racism are inherent to the Black identity.[35] Black people commonly experience explicit and implicit racial biases as well as subtle and blatant interpersonal and institutional discrimination. Racism and discrimination both have consequences for mental and physical health. In particular, racism is accompanied by high levels of stress (which can contribute to other illnesses) and higher rates of hypertension, a chronic illness common in the Black population.[36] Experiencing racism also interrupts sleep, which can contribute to the prevalence of other diseases like cardiovascular disease and mortality.[37] Therefore, race is not a social determinant of health—rather racism is the social determinant of health.

Similarly, once in a hospital or clinic, racism can determine the level of care a Black person can expect to receive. Studies have shown that provider bias, or discriminatory views, attitudes, and behaviors that clinicians exhibit or rely upon either knowingly (consciously) or unknowingly (subconsciously) to treat Black patients can affect how physicians and nurses treat Black patients.[38] For instance, Black people are less likely than White people to survive childbirth.[39] Black people have lower survival rates of diseases like certain cancers.[40] Black people also have lower rates of successful treatment for chronic diseases like diabetes and chronic pain.[41] These examples of racial disparities, in part, can be attributed to their illness and complaints of poor health being taken less seriously by their physicians and nurses. Black people are also frequently presumed to be untrustworthy, drug-seekers, or non-compliant by clinicians. Attesting to this, a 2022 study found that among over forty-thousand history and physical notes from eighteen thousand adult patients who sought care between 2019 and 2020, clinicians were 2.54 times more likely to use negative descriptors like "resistant" and "noncompliant" in Black patients' electronic health records (EHR) than White people's EHR.[42] These negative views of Black people encourage physicians to take their symptoms of illness less seriously and give them poor treatment. Provider bias is rarely displayed through blatant racist behaviors, but rather subtle behaviors and attitudes. But these subtle behaviors and attitudes are part of what makes racism and not race a social determinant of health.

The typically inferior status of Black health is best understood as inequities in access to the social determinants of health. Social research tells us that Black people are less likely to have access to social determinants of health, creating what is known as the White-Black gap in health.[43] So when we talk about the health of Black people as a group, we necessarily have to talk about how their Black identity functions within the social institutions that can give or withhold social determinants of health. Inequities arise when institutions' policies, laws, and regulations unjustly negatively affect Black people while privileging White people. The inferior nature of Black health is created and maintained and thrives upon inequities in the social institutions that control our lives and the lesser value that people who run these institutions place on Black lives. Given how important social determinants of health can be to health, wellbeing, and living the kinds of lives that we want to live, in this book I explore examples of the ways that institutions withhold social determinants of health from Black people and what has to change for a healthier Black population.

Chapter Summaries

Each chapter, including this one, is written as a solo-standing chapter, meaning that some topics such as housing are repeated in multiple chapters, although specifically discussed in relation to the relevant chapter topic. Part of my intention is to make each chapter able to be read and understood without reading any of the other chapters. Of course, to get a better picture of the social determinants of Black health, I recommend reading the book in its entirety.

Each chapter is meant to be an example of how inequities in Black people's lives affect their overall health. I picked these particular examples because they interest me and I hope they interest readers. Additionally, the research, which includes the stories, provides the most compelling evidence that inequities in social determinants of health are contributing to Black people's poor health. I picked the examples of pregnancy and birth, pain management, sleep, and cardiovascular disease because these are just some of the pressing issues facing Black health.

These chapter topics are also personal. I have had my own bouts with cardiovascular disease and have had family members die from the disease. I have also struggled with poor quality and quantity of sleep since my teenage years and once struggled with women's health issues. On multiple occasions, clinicians have not believed my chronic pain until I finally found a physician willing to listen and help. Clinicians have also said and done racist things to me during the course of my care. I cannot even count the number of times clinicians relied on racial stereotypes to ignore my illnesses. I have also had illness interrupt my life and made pursuing my academic and personal passions more difficult. In fact, this book was written (and delayed) while preparing for, undergoing, and recovering from multiple major surgeries. Yet, I feel lucky; I have been afforded many privileges that allowed me to get the care that I needed, despite the hurdles of physician bias and racism. But I know many people are not as fortunate as I am, so I picked these chapter topics for them and myself.

In Chapter 1: *Pregnancy and Birth*, I first discuss the history behind the American government's interest in Black women's bodies, including using their bodies as entities to produce more enslaved African Americans. African and African American women's historical lack of bodily autonomy is the precursor to discussing contemporary Black childbirth mortality, or Black people's higher rates of death during or soon after giving birth.[44] In the case of contemporary Black childbirth mortality, the historical context is the precursor to some of its contributing factors such as clinicians' racial and gender biases and stereotypes about Black women. I also discuss other contributing factors to differing childbirth mortality rates among Black and White people including Black people's inequitable access to health care and Black women's income inequality. I also discuss the implications of "weathering," the biological and physiological effects of social disadvantage, for pregnant people and their fetuses. To illuminate this discussion of Black pregnant people, I also include stories about Black women who have experienced provider bias and obstetric violence while seeking care during their pregnancy. In this chapter I use the terminology *Black birthing people* and *Black birthing mortality* to include any Black person, regardless of gender, that can give birth and subsequently die, however, some issues are specifically women issues. Additionally, we do not have a lot of research on Black birthing people, instead, most researchers use the term *women* because that is the population they studied in the research. So, to retain the integrity of the research and scholarship, I use the terms noted in the relevant research. When appropriate I use the terms *women* and *Black birthing people*, for the sake of accuracy and inclusion.

In Chapter 2: *Pain Management*, I discuss the research on the systemic inequities in health care that act as barriers to Black people's adequate pain management. Research tells us that Black people receive less pain therapy, including drugs for pain, and report lower rates of adequately managed pain than White people.[36] Research on the attitudes and behaviors of physicians and nurses toward Black patients reveals that clinicians' biases are a major contributing factor to Black people's lesser pain management.[45] To ground clinicians' biases against Black people, I discuss the many false beliefs about human anatomy and physiology that have been historically attached to Black bodies dating back to slave physicians' writings on Black bodies. In this chapter I introduce the concept of medical racism and its effects on Black patients' access to pain care. As an additional point of discussion, I use patient testimonies attesting to Black people's individual experiences with nonchalant physicians and nurses who ignored their cries of pain. From this discussion it is evident that there is a connection between historic views of Black bodies and contemporary views, with little progression to seeing Black people as fully human.

In Chapter 3: *Sleep*, I discuss sleep disparities that exist between Black and White people. Black people, on average, get less sleep and lesser quality of sleep than White people.[46] Although income and education levels are a great contributor to this sleep disparity, it is not the only contributing factor given that Black people with professional degrees and high incomes still sleep less than White people who have high school diplomas and lower incomes. This phenomenon is typically attributed to stresses associated with racism and microaggressions that most Black people, regardless of income and education experience.[47] The greatest contributor to racial disparities in sleep, however, is housing, one of the most important social determinants of health. Where a person lives determines the quality of their sleep, and on average Black people, even when they have high incomes and professional degrees, live in poorer neighborhoods.[48] Poorer neighborhoods tend to have higher levels of noise and air pollution, higher crime rates, and less access to healthy foods and recreation, all which discourage restful sleep.[49] In this chapter I briefly discuss some of the history behind US housing laws that pushed Black people into poorer, resource-deprived neighborhoods and how this contributes to disparities in sleeplessness. I also devote a significant portion of this chapter to discussing environmental racism in states like Michigan, Mississippi, Louisiana, and Texas. The environmental injustice that pollutant emitting facilities impose on Black people (and other people of color) and the economic poor demonstrate how social institutions can affect Black people's sleep health and overall health.

Lastly, in Chapter 4: *Cardiovascular Disease*, I discuss Black people's unequal experiences of poor cardiovascular health including hypertension, stroke, and myocardial infarction (aka heart attack). I include an exploration of contributing factors including clinical factors like diabetes, and social factors like stress caused by inequities in access to social determinants of health like housing, income, and experiences with racism. I also discuss lifestyle choices and cultural practices that influence diet, and exercise, while also discussing the social influences on these so-called choices. Additionally, clinicians' biases can discourage aggressive cardiovascular care for Black patients, so I also discuss health care's contribution to Black people's experiences with cardiovascular disease. The literature is rich with patient narratives detailing Black people's experiences with cardiovascular disease and the social determinants of health, so I use them to detail the gender differences in experiences with cardiovascular disease, including risk factors. In particular, Black men have some of the worst outcomes with heart disease out of all the racial and gender groups, and the social determinants of their experiences are worth spotlighting.

Conclusion

For many people stories like that of Hargrove made them aware of issues in Black health that they had never realized. The COVID-19 pandemic has been the wakeup call that many people needed for them to accept that (1) everyone's health, near and far, is intimately tied to our neighbors' health; (2) social determinants of health are vital to wellbeing; (3) racism affects public health; (4) when some people do not have the resources they need to maintain their health, everyone's health is affected; and (5) denying health to Black people is an act of anti-Black violence against them. Although I, like many other scholars, have studied Black health long before the COVID-19 pandemic began, I want to take this opportunity to use the information in this book to capitalize on the momentum Black health is gaining.

My contribution to the moment is this book on Black health. My goal is to make it clear that worse health outcomes for Black people are ultimately injustices and representative of White supremacy wielding its power over Black people. Given the importance of health to our overall wellbeing, I hope readers see what is at stake for us all if we ignore the status of Black people's health. A discussion of Black health and its social determinants is a worthwhile task because inferior Black health creates a paradigm in which the benefits of health, namely wellbeing and social mobility, are routinely withheld from Black people because of their race. Given the data that we have on this unjust relationship between Black people and health and health care, it is imperative that we create a productive dialogue on what it means to be Black and sick in America.

Discussion Questions

1. Why should we care about Black people's health?
2. How do everyday social factors influence our health?
3. Why does racism matter for racial disparities in health?
4. What are some of the problems with biological explanations of race?
5. What are some of the benefits and challenges of a social explanation of race?

1

Why Are Hospital Births Unsafe
for Black People?

Shalon Irving was an epidemiologist at the Centers for Disease Control and Prevention (CDC). Irving had multiple graduate degrees, access to health insurance, and a great support system consisting of family and many well educated, professional friends. Irving was also a Black, pregnant woman.

Long before her pregnancy, however, Irving was treated for uterine fibroids and learned she had a genetic mutation that made her prone to blood clots. She also had hypertension.

After delivering her daughter via C-section she developed a lump on the incision. After a physician told her it was nothing to worry about, her physician diagnosed her with a hematoma and treated her swollen legs and addressed her rapid weight gain. Soon after this Irving had a series of doctor visits and home visits for her increasing blood pressure, swollen legs and her incision wasn't healing. But she was consistently told this was normal.

One night while at home with her mother and child, Irving gasped, clutched her heart, and passed out. While in the ambulance a breathing tube was incorrectly placed by emergency technicians. When Irving arrived at the hospital, she never regained consciousness. After spending four days in the hospital, she was removed from life support and died soon after; all before her daughter reached the age of one.[1]

In the United States, stories like Irving's are unfortunately too common. In America, Black people are up to three times more

Black Health. Keisha Ray, Oxford University Press. © Oxford University Press 2023.
DOI: 10.1093/oso/9780197620267.003.0002

likely than White people to die during or soon after (up to one year) childbirth.[2] In states like Louisiana, the rate is even higher with four Black people to every one White person. While states like North Carolina have used social programs to lower their Black birthing mortality rates, for most Black Americans, if you are a Black pregnant person, delivering a baby in an American hospital can cost you your life. Despite the United States' wealth, health care systems, and abundance of obstetrics and gynecology knowledge, Black pregnant people are still dying. They are losing their lives and leaving children and families behind. This chapter uses stories like Irving's to explore explanations for high rates of Black birthing mortality and what is being done to end it.

When trying to explain why Black pregnant people are dying during or soon after childbirth, it would be misguided to focus on any one particular social determinant of health. For instance, a lack of education does not explain Black birthing mortality rates as Black women are one of the most educated groups in America.[3] Additionally, adverse childhood experiences, like teenage pregnancy, also do not explain Black birthing mortality rates as teen pregnancy among Black girls has significantly declined over the years, but Black birthing mortality has not declined.[4] Yet if we look at how social and cultural determinants of health have historically intersected with Blackness, class, and gender, we get a more complete story. For instance, if we look at how access to health care, provider bias, and historical abuses of Black pregnant people's bodies intersect or how inequities in housing and income intersect in Black pregnant people's lives, we have a better understanding of what contributes to Black birthing mortality.

Some of the social, cultural, and political determinants of high rates of death among Black pregnant people include (1) gynecology and obstetrics' White supremacist origins; (2) medical racism, including clinicians' racial biases against Black pregnant people (sometimes called obstetric violence); and (3) social inequities like those that exist in income and housing access. Lastly, a large determinant of Black birthing mortality rates is "weathering," or the cumulative biological and physiological effects of stressors like social disadvantages. Piecing together all of these intricately connected social determinants of Black birthing mortality, a picture emerges of a preventable, and incredibly racist act against Black people and their families. But first, before exploring the social determinants of Black birthing mortality, it is absolutely necessary to discuss the historical framework behind Black birthing mortality because the history of Black women's reproductive lives in the United States set forth a legacy of violence against Black people who want to bear children.

Government Interest in Black People's Reproductive Lives

Since the day that African people were bought, kidnapped, and tricked into being enslaved and brought to the shores of America, the US government has sought to control how and when Black people reproduce. Its interest was driven by colonialism, greed, White supremacy, or White superiority, which were all supported by pseudo-scientific evidence for Black people's genetic inferiority. These values were demonstrated by slave owners' treatment of enslaved Black women as valuable property. Enslaved Black women (and men) were used as an endless well of economic gain for their White slave owners through their ability to create more children, thus more enslaved people to work for them or to be sold to other White slave owners. This sentiment can be seen in laws like those passed in Virginia when as early as 1662 the legislature passed laws stating that the status of the child would be the same status of the mother.[5] This means that enslaved mothers birthed enslaved children, allowing slave owners to use Black women's bodies to create more enslaved people and more economic gain for themselves. Black women were valuable because they maintained White people's wealth. Overall, controlling and enslaving Black women was a way for the United States to maintain a power system where White people were on top and Black people found themselves on the bottom with no autonomy over their lives.

In the seminal text, "Killing the Black Body," Dorothy Roberts[6] gives an extensive history of the government's interest in Black women's bodies. Using Roberts' historical account of Black women, their lack of personhood, autonomy, and freedom began with the view that enslaved Black women were not really *women* in the same way that White women were *women*. The characteristics that were thought to be womanly like femininity, delicacy, softness, chastity, and a fondness for motherhood were strictly associated with White women but not Black women. Instead, Black women were thought to be hard and driven by their sexual desires, making them sexual deviants.

This sexualized view of enslaved Black women can be seen in the *Jezebel* stereotype, which was common at that time. Referring to the Biblical character, Jezebel, who was controlled by her sexual desires and left men unable to control their sexual desires, became a popular way to characterize Black women. Instead of being chaste like White women they were thought to lack virtue and instead have an innate lust for promiscuity. As Roberts tells us, this view of Black women was used to further deny them autonomy over their bodies. For example, because they were seen as lustful beings who used their nature to tempt men with sex, when White men sexually abused Black women, it was not seen as morally or legally wrong in the same way sexual abuse against White women was seen as wrong. And aided with White slave owners' views that Black women were property, the stereotype that Black women were governed by sexual desires meant that Black women could not be sexually harmed. Even when slavery was outlawed in the United States, the Jezebel stereotype and its effects never ended. Instead, stereotypes about Black women's sexuality continued to shape social and cultural customs and US law, including outlawed interracial marriage between

Black and White people, denying titles like *Miss* to Black women, and not allowing Black women to try on clothing in clothing stores.

When Black people were no longer legally enslaved, the belief among White people was that when Black women gained freedom, they lost the ability to be good mothers who raised good children.[7] It was as if Black people needed to live under White people's control to be proper parents. The Jezebel stereotype encouraged the belief that Black women were bad mothers and procreated without discretion. It also encouraged the false belief that Black women did not care about contraceptives or family planning. According to Roberts the stereotype that Black women were overly sexual led to the belief that the government must impose family planning onto Black families since Black women could not control their sexual desires nor how often they procreated. These ideas were fueled by beliefs in eugenics and often led to inhumane treatment of Black women (and other people).

Eugenics

Guiding government interest in Black people's reproduction was the idea of *eugenics*, or the belief that some traits that parents pass on to their children are desirable and should be a part of the human gene pool and undesirable traits like laziness, lack of intellectualism, or a propensity for criminal behavior are inheritable and should not be a part of the human gene pool. Relying on false scientific evidence for distinct racial groups, eugenicists mistakenly believed these kinds of undesirable traits could be passed on from parents to children and aimed to remove them from the human population by controlling reproduction. One of the many problems with eugenics is that it is racist and ableist in nature. Eugenicists believed that most White people did not pass on undesirable traits to their children. Rather they believed that Black people, eastern European immigrants, cognitively and physically disabled people, and others passed on undesirable traits and, therefore, should not be allowed to procreate.[8] Drawing from discourse in the United States, the concept of eugenics was used by Nazis to justify their inhumane treatment and murder of Jewish people, disabled people, gay people, and others they deemed undesirable. Eugenics was eventually found to be unscientific, but it did an incredible amount of damage in Europe and in America. Specifically, in the United States, eugenics was used to justify racist treatment of Black people.

Eugenics has been around as early as the nineteenth century, but became rooted in America in the early twentieth century when the American government took measures to control Black people's rates of procreation while attempting to hide the eugenics beliefs behind their actions. Public health officials used community leaders like clergy members to encourage Black women to use contraceptives. They also established birth control clinics to give Black women access to birth control. In many instances White public health officials ignored that Black people were already using contraceptives and other family planning tools to control the size of their families. Instead, they believed Black people were too ignorant to control their reproduction and it was up to White people to educate them and in some instances do it for them. Similarly, believing that Black people procreated recklessly and drained social resources, the government also took overt steps to limit Black procreation by lying and deceiving Black people into sterility.

White eugenicists denied that there were social causes for Black people's poor health and thus did not support social programs like those meant to financially support the poor or to offer them health care. White eugenicists did not support social programs on the grounds that they prolonged the lives of people with inferior genes and helped them pass on poor lineage to other people. Instead, public health measures were implemented to severely limit the Black population. For example, Black men in prisons and in institutions for the mentally ill were castrated so that they could not reproduce. And in the 1930s and 1940s, lasting until the mid-1970s,

North Carolina's Eugenics Commission sterilized almost 8,000 adults and children, often because they were poor, "imbeciles" or "idiots," which we would now refer to as mentally ill.[9] About 5,000 of these people were Black. The commission, though, called them "morons" and people "saved from parenthood." In 2002, the North Carolina governor issued a formal apology to the people who were victims of forced sterilization. In 2012, North Carolina was going to be the first state to recognize its abuses and compensate victims of their eugenics programs, but the bill was not supported by state senators.

We can especially see the influence of eugenics on Black people during the 1960s and 1970s when it was revealed that many Black people were given hysterectomies (removal of uterus, cervix, fallopian tubes, and sometimes ovaries) and therefore made sterile without their consent. In an act of deception, the medical staff would tell them they were only undergoing minor surgeries like removing their tonsils.[10] This happened to Fannie Lou Hamer in 1965 in a Mississippi hospital when a physician was meant to remove a small tumor on her uterus and instead did a complete hysterectomy without her consent. Hamer's experiences were so common among southern Black people that removing their uteruses without consent became known as a "Mississippi appendectomy."[11]

Similarly in 1972 a group of medical students revealed that a hospital in the northern United States performed unnecessary hysterectomies on Black people for the purposes of training students. The students also revealed that the hospital performed these hysterectomies but did not record the procedures in the patients' records, performed hysterectomies when safer alternatives could have been used, and that Black patients were pressured into signing forms that gave medical staff permission to sterilize them even though they did not understand the documents.

One of the most notable stories of abuse and stripping Black people of their reproductive rights is that of sisters Minnie Lee Relf, age fourteen, and Mary Alice Relf, age twelve.[12] The Relf sisters were a part of a large family consisting of four other siblings and poor, (formally) uneducated parents who worked as farm hands in Montgomery, Alabama. In 1973 nurses from the federally funded Montgomery Community Action Agency asked the parents if the Relf sisters (and another sister, Katie) could take part in the then experimental Depo-Provera contraceptive, which was delivered in the form of a shot. The agency representatives believed that being poor and Black made them a candidate for federally funded contraception. Although their mother was unable to read or write, she gave her consent by signing an "X" on the consent forms. With this "X" the nurses began to regularly inject the contraceptive into the sisters' arms. The government eventually stopped administering the injections to girls and women once their link to cancer was revealed in laboratory tests. Though, it was too late for Minnie Lee and Mary Alice. As part of the program they were taken to the hospital and underwent surgery to make them sterile without their parents' knowledge.

During the Relf's federal lawsuit it was revealed that some 100,000 to 150,000 poor women and girls, almost half of which were Black, were sterilized under this program. The lawsuit also revealed the level of deception program officials used to get women and girls to take the contraceptive shot. For instance, the officials would threaten to take away families' welfare benefits if they did not participate in the program.

Although the 1970s were not that long ago, there are more contemporary examples of the US government's interest in Black people's reproductive lives. Between 1997 and 2003 the California state prison system sterilized about 1,400 women inmates, most of them Black women, without their consent, often through deceit.[13] From 2006 to 2010 more Black women inmates were also sterilized.[14] In 2008, Kelly Dillion, a twenty-four-year-old Black, imprisoned woman and survivor of domestic violence was in the California prison system for murdering her husband. She told the prison physicians that she had painful cramps and they told her she needed a hysterectomy to treat her cervical cancer. Later, another physician told her that in fact she did not have cervical cancer. Additionally, some people were not told they would be sterile until after they came out of surgery. Other people had hysterectomies without their consent, right after giving birth. In 2014, Dillion and her attorney helped to pass a bill that banned forced sterilizations for the sake of birth control.

Performing hysterectomies on imprisoned people is state sanctioned reproductive violence against Black people and people made vulnerable by their imprisonment. The government's goal is to control Black people's bodies. When the government controls people's reproduction they exert power over how the course of their entire life will unfold. Taking away Black individuals' ability to control their reproduction hurts individuals by depriving them of their autonomy, but it also robs Black people of our humanity; it sends the message that our lives are not worthy of existing. It also reinforces racist stereotypes that Black people will reproduce without regard for finances and instead will rely on state welfare systems if a White authority figure does not intervene. In fact, in regard to the California prison hysterectomies, court documents later revealed that one of the physicians who performed the hysterectomies called them "cheaper than welfare," indicating that he preferred medically unnecessary interventions over the possibility of Black people using welfare services.

The people in these stories are mostly Black, but they are also mostly poor, and mostly women. A thread that runs through these stories, however, is that Black people are made vulnerable to inhumane treatment not because they embody multiple identities, but because racist ideologies that drive White supremacy say that these identities do not matter. Furthermore, White supremacists have elevated these opinions as the ones that matter. Many White people do not see the humanity in Black people that they see in themselves. As such they believe they are justified in treating Black people in ways that they would never accept themselves and in ways they would never treat fellow White people. This is the legacy of believing in *race* as a biologically real concept and not as a social construct. This is also the legacy of relying on race to justify White superiority and thus White authority over other humans. For contemporary Black pregnant people these views of Black people's humanity translate into no regard for their reproductive autonomy, which can encourage little regard for their obstetric health.

So far I have only given a few examples of the US government's interest in and control of Black women's bodies. There is, however, a much more extensive, racist, and violent history than what I have given here. Yet what is important is that this history has created a legacy that did not end when slavery or types of legal racial discrimination (i.e., housing segregation) ended. Instead, the government's interest in Black women's bodies seen during America's enslavement of Black people and afterward in eugenic policies has left a stain on medicine's relationship with Black pregnant people. In many of the interactions Black pregnant people have with clinicians we can see remnants of this legacy. Clinicians' attitudes and behaviors toward Black pregnant people still reflect an enslaved and slaveowner mentality, and this has great consequences for the survival of Black pregnant people. To further examine the history between American institutions and Black women, next I discuss an example of reproductive experimentation that enslaved Black women were forced to endure, giving us some of the obstetrical and gynecology knowledge we have today.

Reproductive Experimentation

It would be a great error if I did not also discuss the violent legacy of James Marion Sims and his contributions to our current treatment of Black pregnant people. Sims was a physician who experimented on enslaved Black women and men during the nineteenth century. For his achievements in experimenting on Black women he is often referred to as the "father of gynecology." Statues of Sims can be seen all over the United States, including at the University of South Carolina in Columbia, South Carolina. There was even a statue of him erected in Central Park in New York City; however, after the city's Public Design Commission conducted a review of hate symbols, it was removed in 2018 and moved to his Brooklyn grave.[15] To not erase the Black women Sims experimented on from history, Michelle Browder created the *Mothers of Gynecology* monument, which was erected in Montgomery, Alabama, in 2021. The monument is near where the experiments originally occurred in the 1840s and near the Alabama State Capitol which still bears a statue of Sims.[16] The controversy over whether statues of Sims should continue to stand, however, continues to be a polarizing issue because of how he got the name "father of gynecology" and who he used to receive his notoriety.

Sims started performing gynecologic experimentations on enslaved Black women beginning in 1845. He would acquire them from White slave owners by promising to board them and treat their gynecological disorders. He would also use enslaved people as assistants. During his tenure as a physician, he invented the vaginal speculum, a version of which gynecologists still use today, and he developed a treatment for vesicovaginal fistula, a sometimes painful side-effect of giving birth.

Sims initially performed his experimentations on enslaved Black women. Some of those women included Lucy, Betsey, and Anarcha. We do not know whether these Black women willingly participated in the experiments, but by their very status as slaves and as property, they would have been incapable of consenting. Even if they wanted to participate in the experiments, if people are owned and their bodies are ultimately not their own, they could not consent without fear of repercussions. In fact, while experimenting on enslaved Black women, Sims would take temporary ownership of them (as opposed to their established owners), giving him free access to their bodies to perform his experiments. Enslaved Black women provided test subjects for Sims because he could buy them and force their participation. In fact, Sims wrote, "There was never a time that I could not, at any day, have had a subject for operation."[17] For this reason I do not refer to the enslaved women as patients, rather I refer to them as test subjects; nor do I refer to his interventions as operations, but as experimentation.

Lucy, an eighteen-year-old woman who had not been able to control her bladder after giving birth, became one of Sims' test subjects. When Sims would begin his experimentations on Lucy, and test subjects like her, he would tell her to get naked and put her body into a position similar to being on all four limbs. Lucy did this while almost a dozen White physicians watched her writhe and scream in pain as Sims performed his experimentation on Lucy's vagina. Sims and other White physicians would take turns inserting a speculum into her body. Sims later acknowledged that Lucy was in great pain and he thought she might die after contracting blood poisoning resulting from his experimentation.[18]

In 1845, Sims performed a similar experimentation on another enslaved woman, Anarcha, a seventeen-year-old girl who developed fistulas after a difficult delivery. For three days Anarcha labored with her first child on a plantation in Montgomery, Alabama. Sims was called to deliver the child, who ultimately died. As a result, Anarcha was left with damage to her vagina, rectum, and bladder. She was also incontinent, and the urine caused infections and pain.[19] She endured thirty surgeries to help her vesicovaginal fistula condition until Sims felt he perfected the surgical technique. After four years of experimentation on enslaved African women, Sims began to perform the procedure on White women, but this time he used anesthesia.

There are, however, at least two ways to analyze how Sims thought of anesthesia for Black women. First, during the course of his experiments Sims did have the opportunity to use it on Black women, but he did not. He did, however, use anesthesia on White women once he started performing the procedures on them. We can think of this as proof that he did not believe Black women felt pain in the same way that White women felt pain. Sometimes, though people will dismiss Sims' treatment of enslaved Black women and say things like "that's just what they did back then." But this argument ignores the abolitionist movement and critiques of slavery that existed at the time. As Karla Holloway puts it, Sims could have chosen differently, but he did not, and "Sim's decision to own slaves indicates his choice between competing ethical paradigms."[20]

Second, there is some indication that Sims knew exactly how painful his experimentations were, how much pain the enslaved women felt, and that people would frown upon him not using anesthesia with enslaved women. For example, when referring to Lucy, he stated "Lucy's agony was extreme . . . she was much prostrated and I thought she was going to die."[21] Sims also omitted the race of the enslaved women when he published his findings in medical journals. Sims even depicted illustrations with "bourgeois white matrons" instead of enslaved Black women.[22] There is a lot of evidence that Sims knew exactly how painful his experiments were, but did not care about his test subjects' pain.

A lot of the knowledge we have about treating gynecological disorders came from Sims' traumatic experiments. Many people today still benefit from the experiments, including his creation of the speculum; however, our benefits come at the expense of the enslaved Black women who were subjected to the horrors of medical experimentation. Harriet Washington states that since his experiments had good health outcomes for some of the people he experimented on and contributed to good health outcomes for some contemporary people of all races, some people may excuse his experimentation as justifiable. Enslaved Black women, however, bore great suffering so that all people with vaginas and all people who give birth can have better medical care. When one group benefits and another group bears the costs, though, this is an example of injustice.[23] Lucy, Anarcha, and the other women and men that Sims experimented on were treated unjustly in a system of slavery that was already treating them less than human. And the injustices didn't end with them; their impact is still being felt today by Black people seeking gynecological and obstetrical care. We see this long-lasting impact in clinicians' biases that act as barriers to care.

Health Care's Biases

Black birthing mortality is preventable; death is not inherent to the experience of being Black and giving birth. Research shows that clinicians' biases, or the explicit and implicit negative beliefs that people associate with some groups of people, are associated with worse health outcomes, particularly for people of color.[24] For Black pregnant people, who are also women, they stand at the intersection of clinicians' biases against women, Black people, and biases specifically directed at Black women. As we explore how clinicians' biases subject Black pregnant people to disrespect and disregard (i.e., obstetric violence), we see that these biases did not spontaneously arise overnight; rather they are directly related to historical negative and derogatory views that have persisted since African people were forcibly brought to the United States and their bodies and families were bought and sold. Although racial biases were once used to justify the violence of enslavement, today, racial biases against Black pregnant people manifest as poor treatment and poor health outcomes for Black people and their families.

Strong and Hardy

The idea that Black women possess "obstetrical hardiness" has appeared in medical literature as early as the 1920s. Obstetrical hardiness is the belief that Black women naturally have the mental and physical strength needed for the difficulties of birthing children.

Slave owners and White physicians believed that Black women could withstand great amounts of trauma so before and during labor they gave Black women very little care. For instance, in 1932 an American physician wrote "the colored woman, because of her lessened sensibility to pain, is willing to endure prolonged labor when a white woman would hours before demanding relief."[25] The literature in the early to mid-twentieth century continued to push the idea of obstetrical hardiness, relying on Black women's supposed lack of significant moaning or groaning during labor, their absent requests for pain medications or other pain interventions. Because of these beliefs, White slave owners required Black pregnant women to continue the difficult work required to maintain their plantations.[26] The belief in Black women's ability to withstand the hardships of labor was contrasted with White people's belief that White women had a delicate nature and because of that nature lacked obstetrical hardiness.

The idea of obstetrical hardiness has not gone away; instead, it has transformed into a new form of biased thinking. The similar idea that Black women have an innate strength that requires clinicians to give them less care and kindness can be seen in the *strong Black woman* trope. When the perception of Black women being strong or "super women" is allowed to thrive in health care, it becomes easy for clinicians to offer them less of their time and attention and to be less nurturing and supportive during treatment. According to Tina Sacks in *Invisible Visits*, less care from providers and constantly being required to be physically and mentally strong for their and their child's survival may be pathways for Black women's poor obstetric health outcomes.[27] As such, the *strong Black woman* trope can backfire; when Black pregnant people die, it can be perceived that they were not strong enough and their death is their fault rather than the hard truth that sometimes they are not given the care they need. The *strong Black woman* trope misguidedly pushes the belief that Black pregnant people are naturally endowed with a strong body and a strong disposition without any attention to how their environments require them to have an outward and inner strength.

Black women are not necessarily naturally emotionally or physically stronger than any other group, and it is not that Black women particularly want to be strong. It is more likely that Black women developed a unique strength so they could endure the hardships of slavery, while also being pregnant, caring for their own children and families, as well as doing the forced duty of caring for White people's children and their families. Their strength was likely never innate; their strength was needed for survival, and it became embedded in their culture. Now, Black pregnant people need a strong disposition to survive racial biases and discriminatory behavior that stands in the way of their access to health care.

The perception of Black women as strong individuals also fails to account for the ways that social inequities force them to be strong. For example, during the COVID-19 pandemic Black women had higher rates of joblessness and housing insecurity than Black men and White men and women.[28] Facing structural inequities like these while also experiencing the emotional toll of a pandemic, all while carrying a pregnancy to term, is difficult and requires a level of durability that to those who are unaware of these structural inequalities may seem innate rather than developed.

Biases about Black women including their obstetrical hardiness, sexual deviancy, or the idea that Black women are hyper-sexual[29] and their pregnancy is physical proof of their immoral, sexually deviant nature, have lingered through the centuries and have become a part of Black pregnant people's public narrative. And health care, despite its typical public image as a noble profession, is not immune to the effects of this narrative and often perpetuates it. Biases are deep-seated in ourselves and in our institutions. Biases become another pathway for clinicians to discriminate against Black people and give them subpar care with deadly consequences. One example where we see clinicians' biases affecting Black people's care is in what should be the simple act of listening.

Listening to Black Pregnant People

In 2018 professional tennis superstar Serena Williams gave birth to her first child via Cesarean section.[30] Soon afterward she began to feel pain and discomfort. She also began to have a very bad cough. Knowing her history of blood clots, she alerted the nearest nurse. Williams informed the nurse about her current symptoms, her medical history of blood clots, and asked the nurse for care, to which the nurse responded that the pain medications Williams was on after giving birth must be making her confused. Williams did not back down and demanded care. A physician eventually performed an ultrasound of her legs, which found no blood clots. Williams, having been treated for blood clots in the past, remained adamant that she needed a CT scan and a heparin drip (i.e., preventative blood thinner), not an ultrasound. Luckily for Williams her determination paid off. She finally received a CT scan that revealed several potentially deadly blood clots in her lungs that luckily had not yet reached her heart. According to Williams:

> I was coughing because I had an embolism, a clot in one of my arteries. The doctors would also discover a hematoma, a collection of blood outside the blood vessels, in my abdomen, then even more clots that had to be kept from traveling to my lungs.[31]

Williams was finally put on a heparin drip. In total, Williams had four emergency surgeries, and her blood clots were successfully removed. Her life was saved. According to Williams, clinicians finally listening to her saved her life: "Being heard and appropriately treated was the difference between life or death for me; I know those statistics would be different if the medical establishment listened to every Black woman's experience."[32]

Williams' story is many Black women's story: one of being silenced by clinicians. NPR and ProPublica collected over two hundred stories from African American mothers and the running theme in the stories is that they feel overlooked, rushed, and ignored during their clinical visits.[33] When Black women report symptoms of poor health, they feel like their clinicians do not take them seriously and are not proactive in their treatment. Despite her fame, wealth, and her White and wealthy husband, Serena Williams, a Black woman, was also silenced by her nurse. Her complaints of pain and shortness of breath were ignored by her care team, and she was made to feel as if her pain was all in her head. Williams' celebrity status and persistence may have eventually gotten her the care she needed, but not all Black pregnant people have the privilege of wealth and celebrity. If Serena Williams was no match for racial and gender biases and the lack of care they can encourage, imagine the hurdles to good health care facing Black pregnant people who do not have wealth, fame, or medical literacy. Imagine how easily it would be to silence a poor Black person who complained of pain or discomfort after delivering a child or a person who felt intimidated by the power structure in medicine and felt they could not advocate for themselves. Receiving adequate obstetric care should not be exclusive to outspoken, wealthy people with celebrity status.

Serena Williams' story demonstrates that often external, systemic factors are responsible for high Black birthing mortality rates. As such, changing individual behaviors are unlikely to make a significant dip in Black birthing mortality rates and give individuals better health outcomes. For instance, typically higher incomes and more education result in better health outcomes for people. But high incomes and more education will not save Black pregnant people from dying during or soon after childbirth. As the CDC reports, pregnancy-related mortality ratio for Black pregnant people with a college degree is 5.2 times that of White pregnant people.[34] Black women are one of the most educated groups in America, yet income and education is not a social determinant for their likelihood to survive childbirth.[35]

One common response to stories like Serena Williams and Shalon Irving's stories is "How do we know they died or were ignored because they were Black?" This kind of question, however, misses the mark. It asks Black people who have data to support their higher than normal deaths to prove the truthhood of the data and to prove their experiences of racial bias, which should not be their burden. Essentially, this question ignores how biases work, especially how biases can influence care for Black pregnant people. Biases in health care can manifest itself in different ways—not listening to Black pregnant people, not trusting their knowledge of their body, and even convincing Black people to not trust their own bodies are just some of those ways.[36] Often these biases are implicit, or subconscious, meaning we are unaware of them. Biases can be so ingrained in individuals that we are unaware of the ways they affect our behaviors. Biases can also be ingrained in institutions like health care. Additionally, our values and our worldviews can sometimes not align with our biases. For example, we can believe that racism is abhorrent or that sexism is unacceptable but still sometimes act in racist or sexist ways. This, however, does not absolve us from trying to rectify how our biases affect other people.

Rather than asking Black pregnant people how they know they have experienced racial, gender, or class bias, we should work to interrogate and correct our personal biases. Some biases are learned but they do not have to be permanent. They can be changed. If we start with the assumption that caregivers have biases, we can ask ourselves "Why do Black pregnant people feel unheard?" and "What effects does this have on the Black pregnant person/patient-physician relationship?" This is especially true when we have evidence that some Black pregnant people take precautions to guard themselves from the effects of biases. For example, some pregnant Black pregnant people will bring a White spouse or White in-law relatives with them to clinical visits to encourage their caregivers to believe their concerns about their health and give them good care on par with the care White people receive.[37] In this instance, they use their White family and friends to legitimize their humanity, hoping caregivers treat them like humans deserving of care and life.

Black people also take other steps to prove that they are deserving of proper care. In Tina Sacks' book *Invisible Visits*, she tells a story about a dinner with her Black female colleagues at the Centers for Disease Control and Prevention (CDC). Angela, a Black pregnant woman at the dinner shared that during a recent visit to her OB-GYN she made sure that her CDC badge was visible to the staff for as long as possible before removing her clothing for the exam so that the staff would hopefully treat her with respect. As Sacks recalls:

Angela quipped that the badge communicated volumes without a single word. It let the doctor know she had an education and a good job that required specialized knowledge of medical terminology.[38]

During the course of the dinner all of the other Black women realized that they all use this strategy. Laughing, they all acknowledged the absurdity of trying to keep their badge on during a clinical visit where they had to remove their clothes. But Sacks says that they did it to show that "we were Black but not poor. That we were women, but we weren't hysterical."[39] By displaying their badges they tried to convey that they were intelligent and that they had good jobs with good health insurance. Their credentials were meant to preemptively address biases they knew they would be subjected to during their clinical visit. They hoped that their CDC badge would prove that they were worthy of great or at least standard care, care not jeopardized by racism, sexism, and misogyny.

Taking steps to appear deserving of kindness and respect from their clinicians like displaying their work credentials or asking White friends to go to their clinical visits is a part of the experience of being Black and pregnant in America. But these behaviors are symptoms of the overall problem of biases in pregnancy care, how those biases are manifested as discriminatory behavior, and how discriminatory behavior affects their health outcomes. Black pregnant people who feel they are on the receiving end of biased care delay when they seek prenatal care, are not upfront about their potential risk factors for illness or death, and do not trust clinicians' care recommendations, all of which can affect their health during and after pregnancy. Our focus should be interrogating our biases and the biases ingrained in the way we practice health care. Interrogating our biases also means trusting Black pregnant people's point of view. They are in the best position to determine if they have experienced racial bias and it is not our responsibility to question them, rather it is our responsibility to make sure that we remove barriers to proper care. Racial biases can be imposed by clinicians, but they can also be just one of the many experiences of racial biases that people experience, which can lead to the social phenomenon that researchers call "weathering."

Weathering

Weathering can best be explained by thinking of what would happen to a piece of paper if it were left outside for a few months.[40] The elements would destroy it. Rain, wind, snow, excessive heat, all of it would deteriorate the paper, eventually leaving it unrecognizable as a piece of paper. Much like the ways that weather can destroy a piece of paper, social disadvantages can destroy a person. Social disadvantages like not having enough money or food or continuously experiencing discrimination can, over the course of our lives, corrode or "weather" our bodies, minds, and spirit, leaving us with poor health. An example of this can be seen in the research on explanations for Black women's maternal health. Research has found that during their young adult years, the health of socioeconomically disadvantaged Black women deteriorates faster than people with social advantages.[41] As a result they can have poor maternal health and a higher incidence of giving birth to babies with low birth weights. Although the general idea behind weathering is that social disadvantages corrode our health, the exact mechanisms are not always agreed upon. The effects of stress, however, are a likely pathway for the biological and physiological effects of weathering.

Stress can cause migraines, backaches, sleeplessness, and loss of appetite. Stress can also impact the heart, blood vessels, and arteries. Stress affects our psychological wellbeing by contributing to anxiety and depression. And for people who already have chronic conditions, stress can worsen those conditions.[42] All people can experience these effects of stress, but Black people have a higher likelihood of experiencing these effects, because of stress-related racism. The stress from interpersonal anti-Black racism like being called a racial slur and institutional racism like being denied a job based on cultural hairstyles or dress can have biological and physiological effects on the body and cause poor mental and physical health for individuals and populations.[43] For example, the body's natural response to stress includes releasing adrenaline and cortisol, both of which increases our blood pressure and heart rate. Race-related stressors are an established contributor to the high rates of hypertension, cardiovascular disease, and mortality that we see in the Black population.[44] Race-related stress provides a pathway to racial disparities in health and explains some of the poor health we generally see among Black populations.

Black people (and other people of color, like American-born Latinx people) tend to have higher rates of exposure to cumulative stressors than White people.[45] Race-related stress is unfortunately a part of "living while Black." Even if a Black person had all of the physical and social resources they needed for proper health and wellbeing, they could still be subject to the social disadvantages that come from racism. This means that weathering is a part of the experience of being Black. For Black pregnant people, in particular, weathering that comes from race related stressors is troubling for two reasons–harm to the individual and harm to the fetus and baby. For instance, the stress from racism and poverty make Black women age faster than White women. According to a 2010 study Black women ages forty-nine to fifty-five are biologically 7.5 years older than White women who are technically the same chronological age.[46] This is because of the cumulative effects of sustained stress associated with experiences with racism. Epigenetics, or the ways that our social environments change our DNA, tells us that stress shortens our telomeres, the DNA structures at both ends of our chromosomes. Telomeres naturally shorten as we age, but certain factors, like stress, can make them shorten faster. Shorter telomeres are associated with disease and shorter lifespans.[47] This means that racism literally kills Black people. Black women are at a higher risk of experiencing the effects of stress compared to White women just because they are Black.[48]

The stressors that Black pregnant people experience are also important because the effects can be passed on to their children as research tells us that the effects of trauma can be transgenerational.[49] For example, trauma from sexual abuse experienced by one person can be non-genetically passed down to future generations of people. Social trauma like racism and the harmful effects of White supremacy and White privilege can also be passed down from Black people (and other people of color) to other generations of Black people, continuing the harm of racism on people who may not have experienced it firsthand.

Black pregnant individuals experiencing stress can pass down adverse health to their fetus. For example, high blood pressure, to which chronic stress can be a contributor, can increase the chances of preterm labor, and low birth weight for children. The pregnant individual's experiences with anxiety, depression, and stress can also cause shorter than desirable gestation time, as well as negatively impact the fetus' neurodevelopment.[50] This means that when Black pregnant people become pregnant, they bring their life's experiences with racism and discrimination to that pregnancy and can impart its negative effects on their unborn child. Therefore, before Black people are even born, we can experience the effects of racism. This also means that weathering is long-term and it is intergenerational; it can affect entire families through the people that birthed and raised them. This also means that racial disparities in health can be inherited, beginning at the earliest stages of our potential life.

For White women, having more income can mean better birthing outcomes, but this is not the case for Black women, adding further support that weathering plays a large role in Black pregnant people's birthing outcomes. Black pregnant people experience weathering regardless of education, income, and access to health care. Even when Black pregnant people are financially secure and employed in stable high-paying careers, they still experience weathering and poor birth outcomes. Shalon Irving experienced the effects of weathering when she would often be the only Black child in her grade-school classes and the bullying that came with it. She also experienced the traumas common to being Black such as death and disease among her friends and family. Irving had access to great health care, great education, and sufficient income, but none of that was enough to combat her social risk factors for dying soon after childbirth. Even when Black pregnant people are wealthy and highly educated, which should give them a social advantage, because they are still subject to the effects of weathering, their health is still jeopardized when seeking proper health care. This means that the reasons for Black pregnant people's higher rates of death during or soon after childbirth is external to them and due to other social factors. Although there are many other social factors, next I will discuss two—income and housing inequities.

Income and Housing Inequities

Many of the stories shared in this chapter are about women with high incomes who have access to many of the social determinants of health needed for proper health and the safe delivery of their children; however, despite their socioeconomic status, racism still threatened their lives. These women's money and degrees were no match for institutional and structural racism. But since Black people are not a monolithic group, I would be doing a disservice to the discussion of Black birthing mortality if I did not acknowledge that not all Black people, in particular Black women, have Serena Williams' income, or Shalon Irving's degrees and access to health care. So on top of racism, many Black people also must overcome other social inequities so that they survive giving birth like not having enough money for life's basic necessities and a safe place to live.

In 2020, on average, for every 1 dollar of income White men earned, White women earned 81 cents and Black women earned 75 cents.[51] Although their wages have been stagnant, Black men still slightly out-earn Black women.[52] Although Black women are one of the most educated population groups in America, the pay gap is the largest for college-educated (Bachelor's and advanced degrees) Black women.[53] College-educated Black women still earn about 35 percent less than college-educated White men; for Black women, more education does not mean more income. Even when working the same jobs, Black women earn less than their White counterparts of all genders. Black women do not make lower wages because they are not asking for promotions to positions that earn more money. Black women ask for promotions at the same rate as White men, yet for every hundred men who get promoted, only fifty-eight Black women are promoted.

Although many Black women have advanced degrees and are employed in jobs that put them solidly in the middle class, many Black women work jobs with lower incomes. In fact, Black women (along with Latinx women) are more likely to work low-wage jobs than White women.[54] This was especially pertinent to Black women's health during the COVID-19 pandemic when many low-paying jobs were also deemed essential to maintaining public life. So when cities went under lockdown and city ordinances mandated that non-essential businesses like restaurants, hair salons, and retail stores close their doors to customers while essential businesses like grocery stores and gas stations could remain open, many of the people who remained working were Black women. Black women were coming into contact with customers at a time when doing so could transmit a deadly virus. Furthermore, the kinds of low-paying jobs they were working were the kinds of jobs that do not typically offer health insurance. During the COVID-19 pandemic Black women employed in low-paying jobs were at a higher risk of contracting and dying from COVID-19 because of the type of jobs they worked and had a higher than average possibility of needed access to health care. If Black women working these jobs did need treatment for COVID-19 and did not have health insurance, they would have to pay out of pocket for health expenses, yet they worked jobs that did not provide adequate income to cover health care expenses. It is also likely that some people put off health care when it was needed in fear of exorbitant health care bills, jeopardizing their health and possibly leading to death. In general, many Black women cannot afford to be sick because they cannot afford to not work their already low-paying jobs. This is an example of how inequities in social determinants of health, like income, can have wide-reaching effects on Black people's health and can cost them their lives.

Individuals' low wages also threaten the lives of the people they live with and those to whom they give care. Black people who work at the type of low wage jobs that raise their exposure to COVID-19 also risk exposure for the people in their home and for their unborn children if they are pregnant. Despite improvement in shared domestic duties among different family members, Black women (like women of other races) are still largely responsible for caring for children and elderly family members.[55] If family members are ill, many Black women cannot afford to stay home and care for them. Given that 80 percent of Black women are either the sole earner, co-earner, or primary earner in their households, Black women's disparate wages means less money and less access to resources such as health care for themselves and for their families.

Inadequate, low wages also make it harder to access other kinds of health care, such as prenatal care. Prenatal care throughout pregnancy can help ensure a safe delivery for the pregnant person and for the child. But not all people have the same access to this necessary resource. Lesser access to prenatal care is one of the reasons for higher rates of Black birthing mortality.[56] In a country without universal health care, where health care resources like medicines and surgeries are very costly, and much of health care is not fully covered by health insurance, certain populations, including people with low incomes and people of color, are left without the care they need, creating racial and class disparities in health outcomes.

Low wages are also connected to Black women's higher rates of housing insecurity. The COVID-19 pandemic highlighted their housing insecurity but it also made the problem worse. During the pandemic as people were losing their jobs and unable to pay their rent and mortgages, Black women were experiencing higher rates of housing evictions. Additionally, a 2020 report released by the ACLU Women's Rights Project and Data Analytics team revealed that based on data acquired from 2012 to 2016 Black women renters had double the rate of evictions than White women renters. In some US states the differences in rates were more than double.[57] Higher rates of housing insecurity among Black women means that they are less likely to be able to afford safe, stable housing for themselves and their families and more likely to bear the burden of poor mental, emotional, and physical health caused by housing insecurity. Furthermore, once a person has an eviction on their housing record it becomes difficult to secure future housing because landlords are suspicious of renters with prior evictions. Sometimes because of a prior eviction landlords will require renters to pay higher monthly rental fees but if a person has an eviction because of low wages or no wages, paying higher rent could be impossible, further perpetuating housing disparities and their effects on Black people's health.

For Black pregnant people with low wages or improper housing, the effects can be detrimental to their health and their unborn child's health. Housing insecurity and low income can be especially traumatic for pregnant people because they have to worry about providing proper housing not just for themselves, but also for their future child. When stable, safe, and proper housing is withheld from Black people because of social factors like low wages, increasing housing costs, or the socioeconomic effects of a pandemic, Black pregnant people are unable to provide the necessary social determinants of health for their unborn child, which imparts a social deficit onto a child that is not even born yet. But housing and low wages are just a part of the story of Black birthing mortality. As summarized in Table 1.1, Black childbirth mortality is also a matter of historical racial and gender biases that still persist in health care, weathering, and lesser access to prenatal care. There are other parts of the Black childbirth mortality story too, including Black women's higher rates of student loans, which make it harder to have income for necessities like housing, food, health care, transportation, and other social determinants of health.[58] Black women are also more likely to have chronic conditions like diabetes and hypertension that may create complications for pregnancy and delivery.[59] Black people also tend to give birth in lower quality hospitals when compared to the hospitals where White people give birth.[60] Overall, giving birth is a risky endeavor for Black people,

Table 1.1 Black Birthing Mortality:
Summary of Social Determinants

- Racial and gender biases
- Weathering
- Low wages
- Lesser access to prenatal care
- Housing insecurity

but it does not have to be. Black people are not inherently more prone to death during or soon after childbirth. The problem is not personal, it is institutional and systemic, therefore, the possible solutions I explore next are also institutional and systemic.

What Should We Do About Black Birthing Mortality?

Higher mortality rates for Black pregnant people are preventable. It is not inherently more dangerous for Black pregnant people to give birth than it is for White pregnant people. Higher rates of Black birthing mortality exist because of racism and inequities in the social determinants of health, which also exist, largely because of racism. The solutions to Black birthing mortality must start at the policy level. First, we can enact state and/or national legislation that targets providers' behaviors and institutional policies that work against Black pregnant people. For example, in 2019 the governor of California signed a bill that requires all clinicians who work in perinatal services in hospitals and clinics in California to undergo implicit bias training. Senator Holly J. Mitchell, who authored the legislation, charges Black pregnant people with asking their obstetrician, "Have you gone through implicit bias training? Because I want to increase the likelihood of my survival when delivering this baby."[61] Legislation like this makes implicit bias training central to properly caring for Black patients. Implicit bias training informs clinicians on the ways their behaviors contribute to Black birthing mortality.[62] A doula and an obstetrician have even published a guide for Black birthing people to help protect themselves from racial bias and for healthcare providers to address their racism.[63] This solution, however, puts the responsibility on Black people rather than on health care institutions to ensure their health and survival, and is for that reason not ideal. Black people did not cause the problem and should not have to solve the problem, but to protect themselves against preventable death, some Black people may want to ask their providers these questions about their training.

Mothers and Newborns Success Act[64] is another piece of legislation aimed at Black birthing mortality. Introduced in 2020, the bill requires the Health Resources Services Administration (HRSA), the CDC, and the National Institutes of Health (NIH) to improve racial, ethnic, and geographic disparities in childbirth health outcomes. The bill authorizes the HRSA's efforts to distribute grants to states for their work in reducing disparities in birthing and pregnancy health, including identifying practices that would improve birthing and pregnancy health outcomes. The bill authorizes the CDC to acquire more data on birthing and pregnancy health. The bill also allows the CDC to offer grants to government health departments to acquire better data on childbirth health as well as grants for campaigns increasing clinicians and the general public's awareness of birthing and pregnancy health issues. The bill also requires the NIH to establish the National Maternal Health Research Network, which is meant to help improve inequities in birthing and pregnancy health and improve health outcomes.

As a part of national efforts to better maternal health in the United States, in 2021, it was announced that as a part of President Joseph Biden's infrastructure legislation, Build Back Better Act, that $3 billion dollars would be dedicated to bettering maternal health.[65] Part of this legislation includes changes to Medicaid that would expand postpartum coverage from sixty days to twelve months. This can be particularly helpful for Black women since they tend to be uninsured before pregnancy, and after qualifying for Medicaid during pregnancy, after they deliver, they lose their health insurance.[66] This new legislation would give them access to health insurance coverage for more time after they deliver their baby. The Build Back Better Act also provides funding for birthing doulas, training for professionals working with pregnant people on how to reduce biases and discrimination in care, labeling some hospitals as "birthing-friendly" if they provide quality care to pregnant people, and other measures meant to eliminate birthing mortality. Specifically, Biden's Build Back Better Act includes legislation aimed at Black childbirth mortality, originally proposed in 2020 by Illinois Representative Lauren Underwood after the death of her friend, Shalon Irving.[67]

Secondly, state and national legislation is one way to improve Black people's birthing health, but implementing policies at individual institutions can also be impactful. For example, quality improvement programs in clinical settings have already shown to help reduce Black birthing mortality.[68] If we required standardized surveillance or requiring clinicians to complete checklists that measure whether Black pregnant people are at risk for adverse health effects and required them to perform screenings, surveillance, or to take further action should the patient need it, providers could make sure that the treatment they provide to Black pregnant people is not affected by bias. Requiring clinicians to provide thorough examinations when Black pregnant people report symptoms of adverse health is another tool to counteract the ways that biases can lead providers to ignore Black pregnant people and delay needed treatment.[69]

North Carolina is an example of a state that enacted legislation and institutional policies that halved Black birthing mortality and lessened the gap between Black and White childbirth mortality.[70] One measure they took was implementing a population health management program, called Pregnancy Medical Home for low income pregnant people. Beginning in 2011, Pregnancy Medical Home is administered via Medicaid and in North Carolina, Black pregnant people make up most of the state's program participants. Pregnancy Medical Home starts with financial reimbursement to physicians who screen pregnant patients for issues that may complicate their health. Physicians are encouraged to screen for ailments like high blood pressure, diabetes, or depression. If the physician identifies a problem, the pregnant person is assigned a pregnancy care manager who helps the person manage their health.

For instance, if a physician determines that a pregnant person is at risk for preeclampsia, the physician might treat them with low-dose aspirin (known to reduce risks of preeclampsia), inform the pregnancy care manager of their treatment advice, and the manager would follow up with the patient, making sure they have access to the necessary treatment and understand why they are undergoing the treatment. What makes this program even more impactful is it helps pregnant people with any inequities in social determinants of health that may get in the way of their health and a safe delivery including access to food, housing, or medicine.

Thirdly, supporting advocacy groups that are already working to end high Black birthing mortality rates can also help improve health outcomes for Black pregnant people. Groups like Black Mamas Matter Alliance (BMMA) and Restoring Our Own Through Transformation (ROOTT) "envision a world where Black mamas have the rights, respect, and resources to thrive before, during, and after pregnancy."[71] They provide resources and educational materials to Black pregnant people, host educational events, and work to shape research and policy that can improve Black birthing mortality outcomes. Organizations like these are led by Black women aiming to meet the needs of the community they serve.[72] Working with advocacy groups gives individuals an outlet to contribute to improving Black birthing mortality, whether that be contributing expertise, time, or money. Supporting advocacy groups like these also supports the people who are already doing the work, people who have cultural competency to work with Black pregnant people, and people who have an established relationship with the community they are serving.

Lastly, as a country we have medicalized birth. We tend to think that all births need to happen in a hospital setting, but there are other safe alternatives like midwives and doulas that can deliver babies at a person's home or at a birthing center. Research shows that doulas can improve birthing outcomes, improve patient experiences, and contribute to health equity.[73] Making more Black pregnant people aware of these safe alternatives is one way to change Black birthing mortality rates. Black midwives and Black doulas, in particular, are trained professionals who offer a different birthing environment and a different level of care to Black pregnant people and they have the cultural competency to work with Black pregnant people and their families. There are some barriers, however, like financial costs, since health insurance typically does not cover the costs of midwives and doulas and these caregivers tend not to accept health insurance, since health insurance companies can make it difficult for them to receive fair and timely compensation for their services.

The importance of alternatives to hospital births became especially apparent during the COVID-19 pandemic. The virus made hospitals an unsafe place to give birth. Since hospitals were also trying to minimize the spread of the virus, many hospitals only allowed people giving birth to have one person accompany them. Not having an adequate support system to be their voice before, during, and after giving birth can be harmful to the Black birthing person. As hospitals had to change their protocols to slow down the spread of COVID-19, births at home or at birthing centers with doulas and midwives became more important than ever before.[74] These birthing environments provided settings that offered less exposure to people and therefore lessened the possibility of COVID-19 infection while providing a safe and supportive birthing environment.

Conclusion

Ultimately, like other health outcomes for Black people, racism and social inequities are responsible for Black birthing mortality. Racism in institutions that control resources necessary for life such as housing and health care withhold proper health outcomes from Black pregnant people and their families. Weathering is the biological and physiological representation of the inequities Black people live with every day and how those inequities affect their health. Weathering is also the mechanism that keeps the effects of poor health running through generations of Black people; but it does not have to be this way. Elizabeth Dawes Gay, of the all-Black-women-led Black mothers advocacy group *Black Mamas Matter*, sums up what we must do to change the narrative for Black birthing people:

> Those of us who want to stop black mamas from dying unnecessarily have to name racism as an important factor in Black birthing health outcomes and address it through strategic policy change and culture shifts. This requires us to step outside of a framework that only looks at health care and consider the full scope of factors and policies that influence the black American experience. It requires us to examine and dismantle oppressive and discriminatory policies. And it requires us to acknowledge black people as fully human and deserving of fair and equal treatment and act on that belief.[75]

Ultimately, we must think of Black pregnant people as worthy of care, compassion, and life; we must think of them as human.

Discussion Questions

1. How does the sordid history of Black women's reproduction connect to present day negative health outcomes for Black birthing people?
2. Why was Sims able to experiment freely on Anarcha, Betsy, and Lucy? Why do we still talk about Sims' "major achievements?"

3. What is the impact of thinking of Black women as "strong and hardy" on their birthing mortality? How do you think they got this label?
4. How do the stories in this chapter relate to the current reproductive health landscape?
5. What is the role of policymakers and lawmakers in Black people's reproductive health?

2

Who Believes Our Pain?

The first time Riya Jama, a young Black woman, experienced debilitating cramps, they woke her from her sleep. She crawled to her family to get help and they rushed her to the emergency department. After waiting for 8 hours to see a physician, she was told that she was experiencing normal menstrual pain and that she should take over-the-counter pain pills. Although the physician told her that the pain was normal, Jama had to be told this several times because she kept passing out. Eventually she realized that nothing would be done to help her pain. Feeling helpless, she broke down in tears.

Jama continued to have similar episodes of pain. She would have extreme pain and go to the emergency room where her pain would not be taken seriously, nor would she be offered a thorough examination. Each time she would break down in tears and a family member would take her home.

After a year of her pain not being taken seriously, eventually a physician allowed Jama to undergo thorough diagnostic testing. Based on the tests she was diagnosed with endometriosis, but by this time, her uterus was severely damaged. After getting her diagnosis her physician told her that her pain levels were similar to the pain experienced when a person gives birth.[1]

Almost all of us will experience physical pain at some point in our lives. Pain, or an unpleasant sensory experience in which the body's tissues are either actually or potentially damaged,[2] is one of the few guarantees in life for all people. There are different levels of pain, and our pain may be concerning enough to seek care from

Black Health. Keisha Ray, Oxford University Press. © Oxford University Press 2023.
DOI: 10.1093/oso/9780197620267.003.0003

a clinician. Once we seek treatment for our pain, however, there are differences in whose pain is properly treated with medications and other pain therapies. Research tells us that Black people do not have their pain adequately diagnosed and managed by clinicians. And they are less likely to have their pain properly managed when compared to White people. A 2012 and a 2015 study found that White patients are more likely to be prescribed analgesics than Black patients for the same ailments.[3] Another 2015 study found that African American children are less likely to receive pain medication for severe injuries when compared to White children.[4] These studies make up a body of research that reveal the dehumanizing ways Black people's pain is treated by American health care. The research tells us that Black people's pain is perceived, diagnosed, and treated differently than White people's pain; their pain is dismissed and diminished, and they are not treated with compassion and concern.

We have the data that shows Black people are frequently subjected to inadequate clinical pain management, meaning they are not given the proper level of medical intervention to not have pain interfere with their daily activities of life.[5] And the largest determinants of their inadequate clinical pain management are clinicians' racial biases about Black people's bodily and mental characteristics, the racist behaviors these biases encourage, and their experiences with institutional racism. In this chapter, I will not debate this. I will not offer another perspective on the violence inflicted on Black people when clinicians ignore their pain, nor will I offer any perspective that makes Black people the root of the problem.

Based on the information in chapter 1, in this chapter it will be a given that (1) racism is a social determinant of health,[6] (2) Black people's pain is poorly managed by clinicians because of racist behaviors and practices, and (3) leaving Black people in pain is incredibly inhumane. Many scientific researchers and academics tend to ignore Black people's personal stories, believing them to not be scientific or scholarly output. So rather than contribute to the systemic diminishing of Black people's lived experiences I will not question the validity of Black people's experiences with pain nor their experiences with racism. Instead, in this chapter I will make extra efforts to highlight stories of Black people in pain. Focusing on narratives about Black people in pain, like the story of Riya Jama, allows Black people to tell their own story and validates what Black people have always known even without the data—health care is abusive to Black people. Black people's narratives reveal the toll this abusive relationship takes on their wellbeing. The narratives in this chapter make us privy to something that is often hidden—the heartbreak, the mental and physical anguish, the tears, the distress, and the hopelessness that comes when a person realizes that the people who are bound by oath and ethics to care for them will not offer any aid because they are Black. This is something the statistical data alone cannot reveal to us.

Lurking behind the emotions in the narratives, however, is the reality of racial bias. Racial biases are a systemic barrier that stands in the way of Black people receiving the clinical pain management they need. Although racial biases are a part of the institution of health care, racial biases are also held by the people charged with caring for patients like nurses, medical students, and physicians. Racial biases among clinicians can be linked to discriminatory medical practices such as prescribing less pain medication or lower grade medication to Black patients than they would to White patients.[7] Institutional racism, on the other hand, maintains racial biases in clinical pain management by reinforcing stereotypes in educational materials. Therefore, in this chapter I use narratives to explore the social determinants of Black people's pain, namely, the ways institutional racism and interpersonal racism leave Black people with inadequate clinical pain management, and how it affects their wellbeing.

History Repeats Itself

Much of how the concept of *race* was used to enslave Africans and justify their supposed inferiority, as described in chapter 1, also serves as the background for Black people's poor clinical pain management. Racist ideology supported the false belief that Black people do not feel pain in the same ways that White people feel pain because of biological differences.

To justify capturing and enslaving Africans and subjecting them to hard labor, abuse, and violence, White people relied on the ideology that the bodies of their Black slaves were different and mostly inferior to their own White bodies. Black bodies were seen as stronger than White bodies, but their minds weaker. Black people's tolerance for pain was thought to be higher than White people's tolerance, but their intelligence was thought to be inferior. Often the support for these ideologies came from White physicians, the articles they published in medical journals, and theological ideals from religions like Christianity. In their writings White physicians attested to significant anatomical and physiological differences between Black and White bodies. White European and White American physicians practicing between the seventeenth and nineteenth centuries (and beyond) were trained to believe in these differences by their medical school curriculum that included so-called scientific facts about the inferior Black body.[8] Slave owners had particular interests in the differences between Black and White bodies because they saw the bodies of their slaves as investments that had to be maintained so they could continue to serve their interests. They often looked to White scientists and physicians for guidance on how to properly care for the bodies of enslaved Africans.[9] This meant knowing how Black bodies worked and the bare minimum resources they needed to continue to make a profit for their White owners through their labor and by birthing more enslaved people.

In an 1851 issue of the *New Orleans Medical and Surgical Journal*, the article "Diseases and Peculiarities of the Negro Race" written by now well-known White supremacist physician, Samuel A. Cartwright, noted some of the differences he believed existed between Black people and White people:[10]

> It is not only in the skin, that a difference of color exists between the negro and white man, but in the membranes, the muscles, the tendons and in all the fluids and secretions. . . His bile is of a deeper color and his blood is blacker than the white man's. . . .

In this journal article Cartwright also noted Black people's different vision, hearing, sense of smell, ability to appreciate music, and position of the head on the body, as well as many other physical and sensory differences. All of his ideas added to the general assumption of the time that on any type of scale or using any type of measurement known to medicine and science, Black people would be determined to be inferior to White people.

Cartwright extended these supposed differences among Black and White people to a justification for Black people's enslavement. He argued that Black people's bodies were sturdy and tough, which was a part of a common *hardiness* narrative in medical literature, which pushed the idea that Black people were physically stronger than White people, almost indestructible. Even when slavery was abolished in the United States, White physicians like Cartwright continued to hold on to their beliefs about the supposed differences between Black and White people's bodies in an effort to uphold the value, and therefore justification for enslaving Black people. Cartwright argued that under the White man's control, Black people were made to labor, and labor made their lungs work harder to oxygenate their blood more so than if they were to indulge in idleness. But with the abolition of slavery, their newfound freedom made them physically weak and ruined their health. In other words, Cartwright believed that Black people were healthier when they were enslaved and freedom made them unhealthy.

A part of the *hardiness* narrative of Black people, encouraged by White physicians, was that Black people were able to tolerate more pain than White people because of their physical characteristics and internal biology. White physicians pushed the belief that Black people's nervous systems were less developed than White people's and Black people could therefore endure violence like being whipped without feeling much pain.[11] Cartwright gave the name "Dysaethesia Aethiopica" to the supposed heritable condition specific to Black people that among other things, made them immune to pain[12] Dysaethesia Aethiopica is another piece of datum that adds to what we know about the historical perception of Black people, their bodies, and their ability to feel pain.

White physicians and slave owners relied on racist ideologies and prejudices to harm, abuse, and commit violence upon enslaved Black people. They believed that Black people were not human in the way they were human, which is how they justified the inhumanity of enslavement. But White people also projected superhuman abilities onto them, like the idea that they do not feel pain, which defied basic standards of human physiology, standards to which they did believe their own White bodies conformed. This inconsistent and illogical view of Black people as less than human, yet also superhuman, did not die with modern medicine; it can still be seen in the ideals that fuel poor clinical pain management for Black people.[13] For example, a 2012 study found that some clinicians think of Black patients as having thicker skin and higher pain tolerance than White patients even though there is no data to support the scientific accuracy of such a belief.[14] Nonetheless, regardless of how wrong these beliefs may be, they are powerful given the control clinicians have over Black patients' care. These wrong beliefs can encourage them to prescribe less or even no pain medication to their Black patients. This puts Black patients at higher risk for experiencing pain, all because of racist beliefs like Black people's bodies do not abide by the same natural limits to which all humans are bound. Given the often debilitating effects of pain and the ways pain prevents us from living the kinds of lives we want to live, leaving people in pain is an inhumane way to treat people. Contemporary scholars have given the name "medical racism" to this kind of discriminatory behavior that occurs in medicine and health care.

Medical racism is the acknowledgment that medicine and its practitioners have been deeply affected by America's legacy of violence and discrimination committed against people of color and that it continues to live up to its legacy.[15] In particular, Black people's experiences with American society, including enslavement and medicine's central role in maintaining slavery, to legal segregation and institutional racism, all continue to shape how medicine and health care interact with Black people. Medical racism acknowledges that racist ideologies, racial bias, and racist practices that Black people often face while navigating health care systems are not a thing of the past but a very real part of our current health care institutions. Medical racism can be seen in all parts of medicine and health care, from certain medical tools working poorly for people with dark skin (e.g., pulse oximeters) to racism in patient care to the racism that many Black clinicians experience from their colleagues.[16] No part of medicine is untouched by racism and people of color, like Black people, bear the burden.

Medical racism explains Black people's inadequate clinical pain management. At least some White people have always believed that Black bodies and Black minds are different from White bodies and White minds. And because of these supposedly naturally created differences, Black people are inferior to White people. In the instance that nature can be said to be responsible for making Black people's bodies superior to that of White people's bodies, such as the case with the *hardiness* trait, Black people's superiority is still used to denigrate their moral status.[17] In essence, their supposed *hardiness* is used as another way to say they are different and not normal humans and another way to perpetuate medical racism. Given their historical roots, racist beliefs like these linger and become a part of the narrative we hold about Black people. Racist beliefs then become a normal part of our society and thus a normal part of health care. The beliefs then become the source of clinicians' implicit and explicit racial biases leading them to make biased care recommendations that do not respect Black people's lives and desires to be pain-free. It is this poor care that contributes to poor clinical pain management and poor health outcomes for Black patients.

Current research supports the connection between historical beliefs about Black people's pain tolerances and their current higher rates of poor clinical pain management. For example, in a study conducted by Hoffman and colleagues, White medical students and residents, who were both responsible for patient care, were asked whether they agree with a series of beliefs about the biological differences between Black people and White people.[18] Some of the beliefs participants were asked to agree or disagree with included the following:

- Black people age more slowly than Whites.
- Black people's nerve endings are less sensitive than Whites.
- Black people's blood coagulates more quickly than Whites.
- Black people's skin is thicker than Whites.
- Black people have stronger immune systems than Whites.

Each of these beliefs are false and have no scientific support, yet about 50 percent of the participants believed that at least one of the false beliefs were possibly, probably, or definitely true. Additionally, participants were given mock medical cases with Black patients and White patients as the subjects and using a pain scale they were asked to rate the individuals' pain. The participants that accepted more of these false beliefs also rated the Black patients as feeling less pain than the White patients.

The false beliefs demonstrated in this 2016 study align with racist beliefs that have always permeated White people's narratives about Black skin and Black people's experiences of pain. For example, in 1913 the White physician George M. Niles wrote, "The epidermis of most Afro-Americans is rather thick, while the terminal sensory nerves do not appear to be normally impressionable, as a general rule."[19] And in 1985, the medical journal *American Journal of the National Medical Association* (a journal devoted to scholarship on the health of people of African descent) published an article that said Black people's thicker and darker skin may protect them from mosquito bites.[20] The false idea that Black people's skin protects them from the pain of mosquito bites, UV rays, heat, and chemicals has always been a part of the collective medical narrative of Black people and their pain experiences.[21] In fact, there is little difference between these historical beliefs and the beliefs participants supported in the more contemporary Hoffman study conducted over a hundred years later, however, these historical articles might be even more troubling since they were published in a journal meant to provide reliable research on Black people. Given how long this narrative about Black people's bodies has been around, though, it is easy to see how it can be used to support the racist belief that Black people can withstand much pain and, therefore, do not need much pain therapy.

Other studies have also demonstrated the wide-ranging implications of racism for Black people's proper clinical pain management. For example, in a 2011 study, Caucasian participants were shown videos depicting hands of African, Caucasian, and Asian actors. In each video the hands were shown being touched by an eraser and a needle. The Caucasian participants had greater emotive reactions to the Caucasian actors being touched by a needle than to African and Asian actors being touched by a needle. Based on their study, the researchers suspected that Caucasian people's ability to share in the pain of other people depends on the race of the person feeling the pain.[22] Studies like this add to the body of research on Black people's experiences with clinical pain management by identifying an additional problem—White people's inability to see Black people as fully human and like themselves. It is easy to leave people in pain or even contribute to their pain if we do not think of them as having the same human experiences as us. Given that most physicians are White, this study shows that understanding how White physicians view Black people is an important component of ending Black people's inadequate clinical pain management. But this also makes potential solutions more difficult because it would require us to reform people's minds, hearts, and more importantly, their sense of justice.

Despite having much more reliable research about how all humans function, how American health care institutions and clinicians think about and treat Black people's pain hasn't changed enough from 1853 to the twenty-first century to end racial disparities in clinical pain management. The similarity in beliefs between Cartwright in 1853, Niles in 1913, and medical students and residents in 2016 show that racist beliefs about Black people's pain tolerance is not a thing of the past; racism still influences how little we treat Black people's pain and how little we care about how pain affects their lives. As I continue to explore Black people's experiences with seeking pain therapy through patient narratives, their stories reinforce that medical racism is still the mechanism that makes their inadequate clinical pain management a norm in health care.

She Must Be Exaggerating

Alexandra Moffett-Bateau is a Black woman who spent many years in and out of hospitals with chronic pain.[23] She experienced unexplainable kidney infections, fevers, and severe joint pain. Routinely, physicians offered her no help and no explanation for her symptoms; they would sometimes send her home with a day's worth of pain pills but showed little regard for the cause of her pain. After seeing multiple emergency department visits listed in her chart, physicians would treat Moffett-Bateau with suspicion and refer her to a therapist or psychiatrist.

After being shuffled from specialist to specialist, and receiving misdiagnoses, a primary care physician finally looked over her medical records. Eventually this led to Moffett-Bateau being diagnosed with lupus. At first, she did not have any problems with physicians or pharmacists treating her newly diagnosed condition while she lived in Chicago. But when she moved to Virginia, she had trouble finding physicians who would properly treat her lupus induced pain. Physicians would refuse to treat her and pharmacists regularly interrogated the legitimacy of her pain. She was often accused of being a drug seeker and denied disability access to her college campus. Once a primary physician even called the hospital where she had been admitted and demanded that the hospital's clinicians not give her any clinical pain management.

One time the pain associated with lupus sent Moffett-Bateau to the emergency department where she then asked to be admitted for further care. After being held in a room for six hours, physician after physician tried to convince her that she did not have lupus and did not need to be in the hospital. After another hour of crying and yelling, and an empathetic nurse holding her hand, another physician came onto rotation, took a look at her, and admitted her with no hesitation.

Racial Bias and Medical Disbelief

As the experiences of Riya Jama (as told in the opening of this chapter) and Alexandra Moffett-Bateau demonstrate, racial bias in clinical pain management can also be seen in whose pain is believed, and medical racism can be seen in whose pain is treated. Research tells us that clinicians often think that Black people are faking or exaggerating their pain in attempt to get drugs like painkillers, which they assume Black people will misuse.[24] Specifically, some clinicians think that Black people perform drug seeking behaviors like crying, moaning, and writhing and contorting their body all so clinicians will think they are in pain and give them drugs. But clinicians see Black people like Jama and Moffett-Bateau through the lens of their racial biases. And ultimately it is up to clinicians, with known racial biases, to interpret these signs and symptoms and determine which are legitimate and which are illegitimate, performative attempts to get drugs. And as an act of medical racism, many times clinicians are more willing to believe that Black people are drug seekers than they are willing to believe that Black people are in pain and in need of care.

Biases also pose as barriers to women, regardless of race, who seek pain therapy. In some studies women's pain was perceived as not as intense as men's pain even when they displayed the same symptoms of pain.[25] Additionally, women's pain was more often thought to be adequately treated by psychotherapy rather than pain relieving medication. Women were thought to have more animated pain responses than men, which when met with gender biases in health care can be the reason women are prescribed less pain medications than men, even when medically necessary. For Black women, who are subject to these gender biases as well as racial biases, and the ways they are uniquely attached to Black women, receiving proper pain therapy is doubly difficult. To get the care they need they must navigate layers of barriers, all while still being in pain. This does not even mention the intersecting biases Black transgender or non-binary people must navigate when seeking pain care.

Jama and Moffett-Bateau's narratives also reveal how Black people often have to be their own advocate to get the care they need, particularly when their pain is not believed and they have to undergo multiple clinical visits to get the care they need. In fact, how well Black people advocate for themselves is an unfortunate social determinant of health for Black people seeking pain therapy. Indeed, it makes receiving proper care the responsibility of the patient and not the responsibility of trained clinicians. For Jama and Moffett-Bateau, both women had to constantly fight to have their pain taken seriously and were continuously faced with disbelief and a lack of compassion. Being our own advocate is exhausting in itself, but it is not the only cost Black people must take on while navigating a racist health care system.

On top of advocating for themselves to get proper pain therapy in the face of disbelief, Black people also have to think about the financial costs associated with multiple clinical visits and other health care costs that occur when they have to see multiple clinicians to get proper care. Prolonged care also requires time away from work, which for some people means lost wages, and the costs associated with care support for children, aging parents, and anyone else they are responsible for providing care. Prolonged care can also cost people time away from family and friends and their hobbies that make life joyful. Black people in pain who experience multiple clinical visits in hopes of getting proper care also have to think about stamina. They are already in pain; do they also have the mental and physical fortitude needed to withstand the anguish of being ignored by physicians? Black people have to take all of this into consideration while preparing themselves to navigate a system that requires them to sacrifice so much just to be believed and treated with humanity.

A 2012 study of Black participants echoes Jama and Moffett-Bateau's experiences with disbelief and lack of care. In the study, Black participants who needed clinical pain management reported that they were met with skepticism from their clinicians. They felt that clinicians believed prevalent negative views about Black people and that acted as a barrier to their care. For example, one participant felt that his clinician believed that he was faking his symptoms:[26]

The medical examiner . . . she didn't believe that it was anything wrong with me. I remember her because I remember

when she was examining me . . . she would look at me like there's
nothing wrong . . . with me and everything I was telling her was
a lie . . . I know that my medical records show everything . . . that
I'm not lying.

Encounters like this are a part of the experience of being Black and
seeking pain therapy. Clinicians have racial biases just like everyone
else, except in their case, clinicians' biases can mean the difference
between a painful or pain-free life for their Black patients.

Given clinicians' anti-Black racial biases it can seem as if there is
a right way for Black people to demonstrate their pain. When Black
people exhibit normal expressions of pain, clinicians can look upon
their behaviors with suspicion. Rather than embracing the varied
and individualistic nature of expressing pain, Black people have the
added burden of presenting their pain in a manner that will help
them be believed by clinicians. A Black person in pain must exhibit behaviors and mannerisms that clinicians associate with typical pain expression and must refrain from behaviors that might
lead clinicians to think that they are faking their pain. Behaviors
like using the restroom or using a phone can often be perceived as
meaning a person is not in *that much* pain. But any behaviors that
are seen as over-the-top like too many tears or too much writhing
in pain can also be seen as faking pain symptoms. Racial biases
in clinical pain management put Black people in the impossible
position of having to find the right balance between expressing
too much pain and not expressing enough pain. They do not get
the opportunity to just think about their pain and getting better.
Throughout her pain episodes and the disruption they brought to
her life, Jama for instance, had to also continuously worry about
whether a caregiver was going to believe her pain and give her care.
Despite showing signs of extreme pain, such as losing consciousness, Jama was still a Black woman seeking care from medicine's
gatekeepers who have known racial and gender biases. Black
patients like Jama are forced to engage in the politics of clinical pain

management, prove their health care needs, and defend their right to care. While in pain they also have to be advocates for themselves, making health care a constant struggle rather than a place of solace.

Another example of how medical racism among clinicians' affects Black people in pain can be seen in opioid monitoring. Clinical guidelines instruct clinicians who prescribe opioids to monitor patients' use of opioids so that it can be determined whether the drugs are helping the patient manage pain and if the drugs are being used as recommended.[27] If clinicians suspect that their patients are misusing opioids or if any other issues arise a substance abuse specialist is consulted. But research shows that when these guidelines are implemented Black people are monitored more closely than White people. For example, a 2103 study in which researchers reviewed records for patients treated for chronic pain at a major United States Veterans Affairs health care facility, they found that pain was documented for Black patients less than it was for White patients.[28] They also found that Black patients underwent more urine tests (i.e., a diagnostic test that can reveal, among other things, what drugs are present in the body) than White patients, especially when prescribed higher doses of opioids. Black patients were also more often recommended for a substance abuse assessment than to a pain specialist when compared to White patients.

This study is the first of its kind to examine racial disparities in how pain is documented for Black and White patients and how much pain specialists are involved in the treatment of patients with chronic pain with opioid therapy. According to the researchers in this study, "The emerging picture is that black patients who are able to overcome the barriers to securing a prescription for opioid medications may still be subjected to differential monitoring and follow-up treatment practices that could impact the effectiveness of their clinical pain management."[29]

The results of their study are a part of a body of research that shows how racial biases lead to Black patients being prescribed opioids less than White people[30] and how racial biases even determine how clinicians provide follow-up care to Black patients taking opioids. Black patients are subjected to more suspicion of opioid misuse and must convince clinicians that they need opioids for clinical pain management. In a society in which governments, clinicians, and public health officials are grappling with over-prescribing opioids and high rates of opioid misuse, Black people in chronic pain are on the other side of America's opioid problems— they are not getting the opioids they need for their health because of biases from clinicians. Some people like Dr. Andrew Kolodny, co-director of the Opioid Policy Research at Brandeis University, see this as a positive side effect of the so-called opioid epidemic— Black people being saved from the health and social problems of the "opioid epidemic":

> Something that we do know is that doctors prescribe narcotics more cautiously to their non-white patients. It would seem that if the patient is black, the doctor is more concerned about the pa-tient becoming addicted, or maybe they're more concerned about the patient selling their pills, or maybe they are less concerned about pain in that population. But the black patient is less likely to be prescribed narcotics, and therefore less likely to wind up becoming addicted to the medication. So what I believe is hap-pening is that racial stereotyping is having a protective effect on non-white populations.[31]

Although it may be true that Black people have lower rates of opioid misuse, this is not a virtue of the opioid epidemic worthy of celebra-tion; rather it's a testament to medicine's deeply rooted anti-Black racism.

He Must Be Crazy

In *Black Man in A White Coat*,[32] Damon Tweedy tells the story of when, as a medical intern, he was assigned to treat a Black male patient named Gary. Gary came to the hospital with complaints of chest pain. He started having chest pains for the second time in a week while working his job at a hardware store. At the hospital he had two normal EKGs and two sets of blood work, all indicating that he had not had a heart attack. He did have high blood pressure though, and he smoked almost a pack of cigarettes a day. Other than that, he did not have any major medical problems before coming to the hospital so the team focused on his high blood pressure.

The team of physicians, including Tweedy, informed Gary that he did not have a heart attack. The lead resident told Gary that he must quit smoking and he agreed. Gary was less agreeable, however, when the resident recommended that he begin taking daily medication to control his high blood pressure. Acknowledging that he had mild hypertension, he told the team of physicians that he wanted to treat it with lifestyle interventions like diet and exercise before trying medication. The team was, however, very skeptical of Gary's ability to change his lifestyle so they pushed him even further. Based on their experience of patients not succeeding at changing their lifestyle they again recommended that Gary begin medication for his high blood pressure. Only now they were beginning to get irritated with Gary's unwillingness to take their advice.

At this point the attending physician took over for the resident. The physician told Gary about his past patients who ended up with kidney failure after wishing they had taken the high blood pressure medication. Gary asked for a month to try a healthier lifestyle and if he could not get his blood pressure into normal range, he would come back and willingly take the medication and whatever else the physicians recommended. Seemingly satisfied with his answer, the team agreed.

As the team left Gary's room the resident asked his colleagues what disorder they thought Gary had. Tweedy thought he was referring to a medical condition, but the resident was referring to a psychiatric disorder. Despite Gary revealing no history of psychiatric disorders, the resident thought he may have obsessive compulsive disorder. The attending physician suggested that Gary may have obsessive compulsive personality. One member of the team suggested that they get a psychiatry consult for Gary, saying, "Maybe if he takes one of their pills, it will convince him to take ours." Despite Gary's astute understanding of his diagnosis and what behavioral changes it would require of him, his discharge summary listed chest pain along with a psychiatric disorder.

Ambiguous Pain

There is an overall problem in health care with adequately treating people's pain. It is estimated that as many as 80 percent of patients in some clinical settings, including primary care settings, have their pain mismanaged.[33] Black people (and other people of color), like Gary, however, are over-represented in these numbers.[34] When the source of pain is not easily identifiable and diagnostic tests do not provide any help at pinpointing what is specifically causing a person pain, Black people are even more likely to have their pain mismanaged. This is also indicative of the difficulties of diagnosing illnesses when pain is invisible versus visible. Additionally, when Black people go to the emergency department for pain treatment, they are also at higher risk for pain mismanagement.[35] When we put Gary's clinical experience within the context of this data, his experiences do not seem unique; instead they seem more like the norm in health care.

After diagnostic tests revealed that Gary did not have a heart attack, nor any other identifiable reason for his chest pains, the clinical team moved on to address other problems. Looking at Gary's story as a solo patient experience we might argue that there was no reason for the physicians to take further action when addressing his chest pain. But if we look at Gary's experience within the larger picture of how Black patients with chest pain are treated on a larger scale, Gary is a part of a larger problem in health care that uniquely affects Black people, particularly when pain intersects other illnesses and disorders that are disproportionately represented among Black people.

When Black people complain of chest pain, clinicians are less likely to suspect coronary heart disease as the cause for their pain than they are for White people, despite Black people being at a higher risk for coronary heart disease and having worse cardiac health outcomes. Black people also receive less cardiac diagnostic evaluations than White people.[36] Given that Gary is a Black man coming to the emergency department with chest pains, and what we know about Black people's inequitable experiences with cardiac disease and cardiac treatment, ideally a racially competent care team would give more attention to Gary's chest pain. But working against Gary is his race, his working-class background, the ambiguity of his pain, and his negative diagnostic tests.

It is possible that Gary's high blood pressure is related to his chest pain. Working in his favor, though, is that high blood pressure can be objectively diagnosed, and treated compared to chest pain, which is often subjective. This is likely why his care team shifted their focus to his high blood pressure. But no matter what tests are used to diagnose a patient, or how objective they may seem, it is people, fallible people with racial biases, that will decide what those tests mean for patients and what treatment patients need. Therefore, the objectivity of tests will not always save Black people from medical racism. Demonstrating this was how the care teams' demeanor changed once Gary did not want to take their care recommendations, reflecting their biases against Gary.

Although standards sometimes change, typically a normal blood pressure is less than 120/80. Gary's blood pressure read 150/100. So, although it was not in normal range, it was not extremely high. His blood pressure was low enough that diet and exercise could eventually get him within normal range. Given this, Tweedy was stunned to hear that the care team thought he had a psychiatric disorder, all because he did not want to take medication. He wondered what made his team think this about Gary:

Given this data, why did they assume that he had a psychiatric illness because he wanted to eat better and drop some pounds before resorting to blood pressure pills? Because he was black? Because he was a patient in a public hospital? Because he worked at a hardware store? Or was it because he challenged their knowledge and authority in some fundamental way? Perhaps it was a combination of all these factors. It was as if Gary had shown himself to be "too smart" to be a patient in this hospital and therefore had to be mentally ill.[37]

Given the ways that identities intersect, when thinking about the care Gary received, we have to take into account Gary's race and class, and how a person with his identities is allowed to interact with health care, particularly at a public hospital, which generally has lesser resources than private hospitals and typically sees more people from lower income backgrounds. All three components of Gary's background and clinical experience are associated with less care, less compassion, and less favorable outcomes.

Tweedy also questioned whether the care team thought Gary was too smart. When Gary attempted to tell them his knowledge about lowering blood pressure and the research he'd done on dieting and exercising, that seemed to anger them even more. They treated Gary as if he could not possibly have enough knowledge about his body and enough education about healthy behaviors to lower his blood pressure. They treated Gary as if a Black, working-class person could not be educated and was certainly no match for their medical education. And again, we have to view Gary's experience within the context of the data that we have on Black people's interactions with health care. For instance, in a study conducted by Ross and colleagues in which Black people from various age groups and backgrounds were interviewed about their illnesses and injuries that required them to frequently interact with clinicians, participants stressed that the clinicians they interacted with assumed that they did not know much about their symptoms or necessary treatments. According to one participant, a Black woman named Ms. Ellis, "The racism and discrimination comes in not listening to what I'm saying. They tend to think that I don't know what I'm talking about. Because I'm Black, I feel that they think I'm ignorant or maybe [they think] I just don't know what I'm feeling, or I have no comprehension."[38] Ms. Ellis' comments about her own clinical experiences seem very similar to Gary's clinical experience. It shows a larger problem of clinicians not seeing Black people as patients who are trustworthy, aware of their bodies, aware of their pain, and able to make autonomous decisions about their health. And in doing so, clinicians continue to do things as they have always been done, at Black people's expense.

Maintaining the Status Quo

Tweedy came to understand clinicians' racial biases through his experiences with the Black patients he treated throughout his career. Gary, for instance, changed the way that Tweedy saw his fellow physicians. Before Gary, Tweedy did not think physicians could racially discriminate against their patients; he thought talk of discriminatory physicians was all talk from academics or about pursuing a political agenda. But when clinicians' belief in medical racism depends on racism being thrown in their face, they put the burden on Black patients to prove their experiences. Furthermore, it leads to the question, "What if clinicians don't come face to face with medical racism? Does that mean it doesn't exist?" And the answer is of course, no. Medical racism does not have to be seen by clinicians for it to exist. This is where they have to learn to trust their patients' word and listen to their experiences with medical racism. But when clinicians do not acknowledge medical racism because they have not seen it firsthand, Black patients suffer.

All people involved in caring for people have to acknowledge that racism exists in all parts of health care for Black people to receive proper care, like proper clinical pain management. Racism in medicine has to be acknowledged at the interpersonal level (when racism is a part of interactions between patients and clinicians in health care settings) and at the institutional level (when the institutions themselves are racist and employ racist practices) if poor health outcomes like poor clinical pain management for Black people is going to change. When clinicians do not acknowledge that Black people encounter medical racism when seeking care, either because they choose to remain ignorant or because they are not taught about medical racism during their training, poor health outcomes for Black people are maintained as the status quo in health care. Their behaviors and attitudes continue a legacy of racism, poor health, and poor treatment by clinicians. If the very people who are the gatekeepers to health care do not believe that clinicians can discriminate against Black patients or that there are structural barriers that prevent Black people from proper health, then there is no way that racial discrimination in medicine and its effect on Black people can ever be eradicated.

One recent example of medicine's lack of acknowledgement of racial discrimination came from a prominent educational and research source in medicine. In February 2020, the *Journal of the American Medical Association* (*JAMA*) released an episode of its podcast, *JAMA* Clinical Reviews, titled "Structural Racism for Doctors-What is it?"[39] The podcast included host Ed Livingston and guest Mitchell Katz, two White physicians and editors of *JAMA* academic journals. Their conversation quickly turned to a conversation about their skepticism of racism in medicine. In the podcast they voiced their disbelief that racism existed because discriminating against people because of their race is illegal in the United States. Livingston also called for the term "racism" to not be used because it makes people feel bad:[40]

> I think using the term racism invokes feelings amongst people, as I just said, my own feelings earlier on, that make it—that are

negative, and that people do have this response that we've said re-
peatedly, I'm not a racist. So why are you calling me a racist?

To publicize the podcast, the journal sent out a tweet on Twitter
with the statement "No physician is racist, so how can there be
structural racism in health care?"

After listening to the podcast and seeing the tweet, many people
were angry with the podcast and those involved with creating it.
Soon after its release the podcast and the tweet were removed and
JAMA's editor in chief issued an apology for the tweet and for the
podcast.[41] Even though they are not directly responsible for the
podcast's content, *JAMA*'s parent organization, the American
Medical Association (AMA) also issued an apology stating that
the podcast was "wrong, false and harmful."[42] *JAMA*'s editor in
chief also live-streamed a conversation with Black scholars who
are vice deans for diversity, physicians, and professors of medicine
and African American studies on the topic of structural racism in
medicine.[43] Additionally, in June 2021 the AMA announced that
JAMA's editor in chief would step down from his position.[44]

This podcast and the resulting fallout for *JAMA* is an example
of how Black people's poor health outcomes are upheld as the
norm in medicine and contributing factors like racism are ignored.
Furthermore, the podcast is one of the many examples of how white
supremacy is maintained by powerful institutions in medicine who
profess liberal values like equality.[45] Medical journals, which are
meant to educate medical professionals and share medical research,
often publish false or misguided information on race and medical
racism that is harmful to Black people. For example, during the
COVID-19 pandemic that began in 2020, top medical journals
published articles attributing higher rates of COVID-19 death in
African American people to a gene that controls the development
of their nasal passage, articles claiming that pulse oximeters, which
don't work as well on people with darker skin, is not a matter of
structural racism because machines can't exhibit bias, and an article

claiming that programs meant to increase diversity in medicine will produce bad physicians. Although these articles are on different topics, they have the same common problem of ignoring medical racism, ignoring Black people's lesser access to social determinants of health, and instead blaming poor health outcomes on Black people's biology or their cultural behaviors. When articles like these are published it makes it even harder to correct Black people's poor health outcomes, making their poor health an unchallenged norm in America.

Another barrier to bettering Black people's health is that top journals in medicine often do not publish articles on race or racism at all. In a 2021 study of the leading journals in medicine, researchers found that from 1990 to 2020, not many articles were published on racism.[46] They looked at top, well respected and well-known journals including *JAMA* and the *New England Journal of Medicine*, among others. Only during 2020 did journals begin to publish viewpoint or opinion articles on race and racism and rarely were the articles evidence-based studies on institutional racism. This 2021 study builds upon studies like a 2018 study that found between the years 2002 and 2015 only twenty-five articles mention institutional racism in the title or abstract in the top fifty public health journals.[47]

The researchers of both the 2018 and the 2021 studies concluded that this obvious blind spot in our top medical journals is problematic for many reasons.[48] For one, a lack of research on race in these top journals, despite documented research on the impact of institutional racism, point to structural problems in medicine. Namely that people in positions of power in medicine preserve their power by uplifting ideas that maintain their power, or the status quo, and suppressing those ideas, like medical racism, that would challenge their power. Secondly, not publishing articles on documented racism in medicine leads to the idea that racism in medicine and its effects on people of color is not important and not worthy of scientific investigation. Thirdly, it fosters ignorance among clinicians about racism in medicine. If we want to eradicate inequities in health, we have to name institutionalized racism as a problem in public health research.

Critics say that the *JAMA* podcast fiasco exposed a long-standing issue with racism in medicine, further revealed by the false or lack of information on race published in top medical journals.[49] When medical journals, podcasts, and other outlets that produce and distribute medical knowledge produce false information on race, they contribute to an overall violent dynamic between health care and Black patients, in which clinicians do not know how to properly care for Black people, they do not acknowledge structural barriers to proper health that are unique to Black people, and instead commit behaviors that harm Black people. Medical journals are supposed to be sources of knowledge that benefit medicine, the people that practice it, and the people that need it for their wellbeing. Instead, our top medical journals contribute to poor health outcomes for Black people and they contribute to clinician biases that leave Black patients in pain.

Another example of misguided sources of medical information about race and medicine can be seen in the content of the nursing textbook *Nursing: A Concept-Based Approach to Learning*. In 2017 the Pearson publishing company removed the nursing textbook from sales after it received negative public reception in response to its statements about how people from different racial, ethnic, and religious backgrounds experience pain.[50] According to the $235 textbook:

- Hispanics may believe that pain is a form of punishment and that suffering must be endured if they are to enter heaven.
- Jews may be vocal and demanding of assistance.
- Native Americans may prefer to receive medications that have been blessed by a tribal shaman.
- Blacks often report higher pain intensity than other cultures.
- Indians who follow Hindu practices believe that pain must be endured in preparation for a better life in the next cycle.

Pearson's president for global product development eventually released a video apology:

> In an attempt to have nursing students think through the many facets of caring for their patients, we reinforced a number of stereotypes of a number of ethnic and religious groups. It was wrong. We should have been more thoughtful about the information we put into our curriculum.

Although this textbook does not include information about false biological differences between White people and Black people like the textbooks of the seventeenth, eighteenth, and nineteenth centuries, this modern textbook still includes false information grounded in assumptions and stereotypes. Often people will respond that these are not racist remarks, but rather cultural norms about social groups. But relying on cultural norms to guide overall behavior towards a social group, especially when that behavior contributes to their lesser access to resources like clinical pain management, those behaviors are no better than racism. Furthermore, the textbook does not teach nursing students the proper way to engage with individual patients, specifically patients of color. Instead of teaching them to trust the patient, engage with the patient in a culturally sensitive manner, and aid the patient's treatment of pain, it reinforces stereotypes that reinforce racial biases and medical racism.

This textbook is an example of how the very sources of information that clinicians use to educate themselves on how to treat patients can be a barrier to ending Black people's poor clinical pain management. And this is how the status quo in medicine— mismanaging Black people's pain—is maintained. Rather than challenging stereotypes to better Black people's clinical pain management experiences, learning materials like this textbook make misinformation and stereotypes about Black people a standard part of the ways we practice medicine and teach medicine to future clinicians who then continue to maintain the status quo in health care. When learning materials reproduce information used to poorly treat Black people, the learning materials themselves become a means of upholding structural racism in medicine. Only by challenging the ways we have practiced and taught medicine and a willingness to do things differently, even if difficult, can we treat Black people's pain in a way that upholds, rather than denigrates their dignity.

Why Does It Matter?

Pain has a multitude of effects on people, from how their bodies function, to how their relationships function, to how much they are satisfied with their lives. As such, how well we manage Black people's pain matters in so many different ways to the person in pain. For one, living with pain can stop us from living the kinds of lives we deem desirable or force us to adapt and change our expectations for our lives. Pain can change the ways we engage with our hobbies, jobs, and other things that we think make our life worth living. Pain has great economic costs too, including the cost of health care like surgeries, medications, and therapy. These costs are particularly high for people who either do not have health insurance or do not have very good health insurance. Even with great health insurance, health care still costs a lot of money.

Pain can also have personal costs to individuals. It can lessen the likelihood of completing higher education and make it more difficult to maintain relationships with our family, friends, and pets. The effects of pain can also contribute to a lack of self-esteem as a person diagnosed with fibromyalgia syndrome noted:

> I don't have the satisfaction of a paycheck or of having done a job well. My home is my career, and I feel a failure at that. I feel like a burden to my husband and family, and I feel useless. Self-esteem is a real problem for me.[51]

Pain can challenge how we view ourselves and how we view our place within our families and our communities.

For most people, the experience of pain is not pleasant. But the actual feeling of pain is but one part of the experience. Pain is also associated with adverse health like depressive symptoms.[52] And because Black people have lower rates of proper clinical pain management, they are also more likely to be subjected to adverse health induced by their experiences with pain. For instance, pain can cause pain-related disability.[53] Black people have high rates of pain-related disability in addition to their overall high rates of disability.[54] Poor clinical pain management has many consequences for Black people beyond just the experience of pain given their high rates of poor health outcomes in almost every measure of health.

Mortality is another example of adverse health associated with pain.[55] For instance, experiencing pain is associated with higher rates of mortality, including higher rates of dying by suicide.[56] And as of 2019, per every 100,000 deaths in the United States, Black people had the most deaths with 870 deaths, while White people had 736 deaths, and Hispanic people had 523 deaths.[57] As of June 2020 life expectancy for Americans was on average seventy-seven years. Because of the deaths and disabilities caused by the COVID-19 pandemic, however, life expectancy for all Americans dropped by one year. For Black people, though, 2020 had a worse effect on their life expectancy. Even before the pandemic Black people had a lower life expectancy, but the gains they made over the years were erased with the spread of the COVID-19 pandemic. Black people had higher rates of COVID-19 infections (1.1 times that of White people), hospitalizations (2.9 times that of White people), and deaths (1.9 times that of White people), when adjusting for age.[58] All which contributed to their life expectancy being the lowest it's been since 2006, eventually dropping to seventy-two years, which is five fewer years than the average. The pandemic specifically lowered life expectancy for Black men. Even before the pandemic, Black men had the lowest life expectancy among all populations in the United

States, but after just six months of the COVID-19 pandemic, Black men lost three years, while White men lost eight-tenths of a year in life expectancy.[59] Researchers expect the COVID-19 pandemic to continue to undo years of progress made in this area of Black health.[60]

Poor clinical pain management doubles down on Black people's poor health outcomes, like those that were created and worsened by the COVID-19 pandemic. When anyone is subjected to pain and poor clinical pain management, they can have related adverse health. But when Black people are subjected to pain and poor clinical pain management, the adverse effects of pain are imposed on Black people in addition to the risks to their health imposed by other racial disparities in health outcomes like higher rates of disability and higher rates of mortality.

Conclusion

Black people's poor clinical pain management is rooted in historical views of Black people's bodies. These racist and sometimes illogical views just never really went away. Instead, they festered and treating Black people in inhumane ways was allowed to become the norm in health care delivery. We have the data that tells us Black people experience poor clinical pain management, suspicion of drug-seeking behaviors and drug misuse. But it is the stories and testimonies from Black people that reveal the toll poor management takes on our emotional, psychological, financial, and physical wellbeing.

Black people's stories tell us that when their pain is more mismanaged than White people a happy life, a life of wellbeing consisting of the relationships and activities that make our life our own are disproportionately withheld from Black people. Their stories also tell us that Black people are in pain simply because of medical racism and the lack of value clinicians' place on their pain free lives. Even though we have to take into account cultural considerations such as the ways that Black people are socialized to endure pain as a matter of stoicism or gender roles, in many instances Black people are not in pain because of lifestyle choices or a lack of compliance with their clinicians' care recommendations. Black people can do everything right but because of racial biases in medicine, their actions and behaviors mean little when faced with clinicians who see no value in Black lives. To end poor clinical pain management for Black people, we have to give equal attention to interpersonal racism like which is exhibited by some clinicians, and structural racism, like the education materials that teach clinicians incorrect information. We have to make concerted efforts to confront medical racism. If we do not, Black people will continue to suffer, and health care will be another institution that further marginalizes an already marginalized population.

Discussion Questions

1. What are some other ways that pain affects the way we live our lives? Do your answers influence how you view inequities in Black people's clinical pain management?
2. What can clinicians do to contribute to a more equitable treatment of pain? How do your answers specifically apply to Black people?
3. What is the relationship between clinician bias and Black people's lower rates of clinical pain management?
4. What are some of the structural barriers to proper clinical pain management for Black people?
5. How can we hold medical organizations like the *JAMA* podcast and journals accountable for their contributions to institutional racism?

3

Is Cardiovascular Disease a Part
of the Black Experience?

John Singleton was a Black man, popular for being an award-winning film director. He was the youngest person and the first African American person nominated for an Oscar in the category of best director for the 1991 film "Boyz n the Hood."[1] He also won directing awards for the 2006 film "Four Brothers" and the 2017 television series "The People vs. O.J. Simpson: American Crime Story."[2] In April 2019, at the age of 51, Singleton had a stroke; two weeks later he died. Likely contributing to his stroke was his struggle with hypertension.[3]

Dr. Clyde Yancy, a cardiologist, past president of the American Heart Association, and a Black man, lost his nine aunts and uncles, and his father to cardiovascular disease and the only condition they had was hypertension. His message is to "Check your blood pressure. That's a hard stop. That's the takeaway; and especially if you're an African American man, check it today."[4]

Cardiovascular disease is the leading cause of death for most gender and racial groups around the world.[5] Every year an estimated 647,000 Americans die from cardiovascular disease.[6] Although from 1999 to 2017 the number of deaths from cardiovascular disease was on the decline for most racial groups, cardiovascular disease continues to be a more deadly disease for Black people. For instance, Black people tend to develop cardiovascular disease at an earlier age than White people[7] and have higher rates of mortality from the disease.[8] Black people are also two times more likely than

Black Health. Keisha Ray, Oxford University Press. © Oxford University Press 2023.
DOI: 10.1093/oso/9780197620267.003.0004

White people to have a stroke and they have higher rates of myocardial infarction, also known as a heart attack.[9] Additionally, about 58 percent of Black people have experienced hypertension compared to 47 percent of all American people.[10] In fact, Black Americans have the highest rate of hypertension in the world.[11] This was particularly important during the COVID-19 pandemic because hypertension also made people more vulnerable to infection.[12]

With about half of all American Black people developing some form of cardiovascular disease in their lifetime, the medical community continues to devote resources to explaining rates of cardiovascular disease among Black people in hopes of developing effective interventions.[13] Although some researchers believe that there may be some unknown contributing factors to Black people's rates of cardiovascular disease, disparities in clinical factors are known contributors.[14] It is established knowledge that Black people's higher rates of uncontrolled hypertension, diabetes, and obesity contribute to their experiences with cardiovascular disease.[15] But why do Black people have disproportionate experiences of these clinical risk factors? How do they shape their experience with cardiovascular disease? At least one answer is racial disparities in social determinants of health. Social determinants of health like poverty, stress from racial discrimination, and unsafe and resource-deprived neighborhoods are contributors to Black people's rates of cardiovascular disease, in general, because they make people sick and make it harder to get care for our sickness.

Unhealthy lifestyle behaviors like smoking, little to no physical activity, and having unhealthy diets can also contribute to Black people's experiences with cardiovascular disease and its clinical factors. When considering lifestyle behaviors' impact on Black people's poor cardiovascular health, however, we must evaluate their behaviors within the context of their access to social determinants of health. When people have lesser access to stores that sell healthy and affordable foods, lesser access to public recreation areas, and higher rates of working multiple jobs, the choices that are available to them are often limited by social and political forces beyond their control. Therefore, in this chapter, Black people's poorer cardiovascular health will be examined within the context of their inequitable access to social determinants of health. This discussion is not meant to remove agency from Black people, nor to deny that Black people can make bad decisions for their health just like anyone can. Instead, my aim is to add context to how lifestyle choices and cultural habits can be influenced by outside factors.

In this chapter I situate Black people's rates of cardiovascular disease within the social and cultural determinants of health. This includes racial disparities in cardiovascular health care. For instance, people of color with Acute Coronary Syndrome (ACS) are at greater risk of death from ACS than White people, yet people of color are less likely to receive treatments like angiography or percutaneous coronary intervention.[16] Along with the social context of Black people's rates of cardiovascular disease, in this chapter I also explore how racial disparities in health care affect Black people's experiences with cardiovascular disease. I also discuss gender differences in rates of cardiovascular disease among Black men and Black women. Although I do not subscribe to a binary view of gender, all available research on gender differences in cardiovascular disease utilizes only two genders and there are some significant differences in typical experiences of cardiovascular disease and its social determinants among Black women and men that are necessary to our discussion. Therefore, I discuss Black women and Black men. Lastly, this chapter ends with a discussion of actions we can take to better Black people's cardiovascular health, including ensuring more access to primary care physicians, and relying on racially concordant care, or when a physician of a particular race, in this case Black, is matched with a patient of the same race. The goal of this chapter is to explore the social causes of Black people's rates of cardiovascular disease and what we can do to change it.

Clinical Risk Factors and Lifestyle Choices

On a rare occasion, Angela Crenshaw, a thirty-seven-year-old Black woman, decided to go into work on a day she would normally work from home.[17] After about an hour at work she felt faint, had difficulty breathing, and had a hard time moving her arm. By the time she went to get help from co-workers, her speech was slurred. A co-worker called paramedics and once at the hospital an MRI showed that there was a clot stopping blood flow to her brain; Crenshaw had a stroke.

After the stroke, Crenshaw had to relearn how to talk and how to write her name. She also had to relearn how to eat, walk, brush her teeth, and bathe herself because the stroke damaged her fine motor skills. Although Crenshaw exercised, ate a healthy diet, and did not smoke, physicians did not know what caused her stroke. Eventually, Crenshaw's condition improved and she was able to return to work and resume some of her typical functioning. After her stroke, Crenshaw wanted to bring awareness to the fact that younger people can have strokes. She especially wanted people of color to be aware of their risks.

Like Crenshaw, when compared to White people, Black people are more at risk for strokes at an early age, even when there are no apparent risk factors. Although Crenshaw did not have any of the known clinical risk factors, heredity, hypertension, obesity, diabetes, and high cholesterol are some clinical contributors to cardiovascular disease. Black people have a high risk for cardiovascular disease partially because they have a high risk for these diseases and ailments.

For example, diabetes is a known contributor to cardiovascular disease and Black people (along with Indigenous and Latinx people) are more likely to have diabetes than White and Asian people.[18] Specifically, Black people are 60 percent more likely to be diagnosed with diabetes than White people and they have one of the highest death rates from diabetes, with only Indigenous people having a slightly higher death rate from diabetes.[19] Diabetes is also very disabling for Black people. For instance, Black people have their lower limbs amputated as a result of diabetes complications about three times that of White people.[20] Their rate of limb amputation also raises questions about when they seek care, the barriers they face to seeking care, and the kind of care recommendations they receive from health care providers once they do seek care for diabetes. Black people's experiences with diabetes also lead to overarching questions about why Black people have such deadly and disabling diabetes outcomes in the first place. And how does their experiences with diabetes reach the point that it influences their experiences with cardiovascular disease? The answer may partially lie in *lifestyle choices*, or what I like to think of as life's circumstances that shape the choices available to us. Unfortunately, too often life's circumstances overwhelmingly end with Black people having fewer choices that lead to healthy lives and more choices that lead to them being sicker than most people.

Choices v. Circumstances

Unhealthy diets, smoking, physical inactivity, and excessive alcohol use put people at risk for cardiovascular disease. Black people tend to have a more inactive and sedentary lifestyle than most other racial groups.[21] And although Black people do not have particularly high rates of smoking tobacco when compared to White people and Indigenous Americans,[22] they do have high rates of being exposed to second hand smoke, with their exposure being double that of White people and Latinx people.[23]

Researchers often call behaviors like smoking, diet, and physical activity, *lifestyle choices*. As the argument goes, poor lifestyle choices contribute to Black people's higher rates of cardiovascular disease, including those clinical factors like diabetes that increase their chances of cardiovascular disease. At least in some instances, actions like eating unhealthy foods are active choices that people make. Sometimes we have the time, financial resources, and nutrition education to choose healthier food options, and we still choose unhealthy foods. But this is not always the case. To make proper choices we must have the proper resources to allow us to choose what is good for us. For example, we must have enough money to buy quality foods if we want to eat healthy since healthy foods can often be more expensive than high calorie, high fat, and low nutritional value foods. In the instance when people do not have enough money to buy healthy food and instead choose unhealthy foods, it is not so much a lifestyle choice to eat unhealthy but more of a matter of circumstances. In many instances, *lifestyle choices* are better understood as *life's circumstances*—bad circumstances give way to bad or worse choices and good circumstances give way to good or better choices. Therefore, when linking poor lifestyle choices to cardiovascular disease, it is more accurate to link cardiovascular disease to a lack of access to social determinants of health, like income and food availability. A fair assessment of Black people's lifestyle choices and how they contribute to cardiovascular disease includes an assessment of the social, economic, and sometimes even cultural conditions under which they are making their lifestyle choices. This includes cultural influences on Black people's diet and physical activity.

Soul Food and Diets

There are cultural considerations that we have to take into account when discussing Black people's experiences with cardiovascular disease. For instance, "soul food," is food that is tied to Black culture and enslaved African and African-American ancestors, mostly from the southern states.[24] Soul food tends to be salty, fried, buttery, and high in calories and fat. The food and methods of cooking food in our cultural diets can be traced back to the way our enslaved ancestors ate. Enslaved Black people were given scraps and undesirable parts of animals for food that had little nutritional value. And often the only vegetables available were the ones that they could grow themselves.[25] Many enslaved people did not have access to a variety of vegetables, fruits, and other healthy foods; they ate what they had and they cooked it in the ways that provided sustenance. Slaveowners were not particularly keen on providing healthy food; they were only interested in enslaved Black peoples' diet in so far as it kept them healthy enough to continue their enslaved labor. As such, what enslaved Black people ate was hardly what we would call completely healthy by today's standards, but it kept them alive, it kept them functioning, and created shared community and culture.

When the legal enslavement of African Americans in the United States ended, many Black people were forced to retain many of these ways of eating because, although free, Black people were still heavily governed by laws telling them where they could, live, work, shop, and go to school. This affected the kind of jobs they could get and how much money they could afford to spend on food. Although many of Black people's current dietary practices have changed as our access to foods and nutrition education has expanded, dietary practices are cultural and people typically retain at least some of the roots of their culture, even as time passes. But food is still communal for Black people; it is celebratory and a connection to past generations. And many of the dishes that were once created out of scraps are now foods associated with community and comfort. Cultural dietary practices are especially important since they are sometimes the only link African Americans have to their ancestors since slavery wiped out much of our knowledge of our histories and lineages. So when we discuss cardiovascular disease and Black people's diets as a contributing factor we have to have a bit of cultural competency and cultural humility. First, if physicians and nutritionists want to counsel Black people on eating habits, they have to make sure that Black people know about the nutritional makeup of their cultural foods and how it can contribute to poor cardiovascular health. Without knowledge about their dietary practices we cannot expect people to make better choices. Second, clinicians must know the social and historical context behind Black people's diets. Last, they must take into consideration the importance of food to Black culture and the ways culture can be tied to identity.

Physical Activity

Another example of the relationship between lifestyle choices, cardiovascular disease, and social determinants of health can be seen in physical activity. As noted before, a lack of physical activity can contribute to cardiovascular disease. Even when we factor in socioeconomic status, a lack of physical activity is more prevalent among Black women (40%) and Black men (24%) compared to White women (23%) and White men (13%). Furthermore, Black women experience greater decline in activity as they age compared to White women.[26]

There are many reasons for a lack of physical activity that are directly related to people's access to resources. For instance, Black people are slightly more likely than White people, and significantly more likely than Asian and Latinx people to have multiple jobs.[27] Working multiple jobs takes up a lot of a person's time and if they have domestic duties such as taking care of their home and children or perhaps elderly parents, there is not much time in the day left for exercise, recreation, or even sleep (which we know also contributes to a cardiovascular disease). For some people, physical activity may be seen as less important than working the multiple jobs needed to provide food and housing for themselves and their family. People may also value using their limited time for sleep rather than physical activity. Other than time, physical activity also requires access to resources such as places for recreation like parks, playgrounds, or gyms that people's incomes or neighborhoods may not allow for.

As such, when we talk about a lack of physical activity among Black people we also have to discuss the employment, neighborhood, and domestic barriers they face that prevent adequate physical activity.

Our health is intertwined with our cultural identities. For instance, some cultural foods that lack nutritional value and a lack of exercise are linked to diabetes, which is a contributor to cardiovascular disease. And some Black people face barriers to eating well and exercising that are also directly related to their oppressive history in America, for instance living in neighborhoods that are not safe for outdoor exercise. If Black people are less likely to have access to what they need to stave off disease, then their limited access to resources and not their lifestyle choices ought to be the target of our concern. If we want Black people to make better eating choices, then we have to give them the resources needed to make better eating and physical activity choices as well as not erase their cultural practices. If they do not have these resources, then poor habits are not always lifestyle choices but circumstances thrust upon them that they have to navigate the best they know how. This is especially true when Black people have to navigate a lack of resources on top of being predisposed to cardiovascular disease based on family history.

Heredity

After having chest pains for two months, Beverly Buchanan underwent open-heart surgery to address blockage in her main coronary artery.[28] Blockage in coronary arteries can cause a heart attack and since Buchanan had a history of high cholesterol and hypertension, she pushed her cardiologist to run tests to determine her health status. She also asked her physician to run tests because she has a family history of cardiovascular disease. Her father died at fifty-eight after three heart attacks, her mom had open heart surgery, and her son also had open-heart surgery at five-and-a-half months old. Despite her family history, knowing that it does not seal her fate, Buchanan also tries to eat a healthy diet and exercises regularly.

Heredity, or when traits are passed down from one family member to another genetic family member, sometimes called family history, can be a factor in Black people's experiences of cardiovascular disease. People whose close family members like their biological parents, siblings, and grandparents have cardiovascular disease are more likely to have cardiovascular disease themselves.[29] Since Black people have a high incidence of cardiovascular disease, it follows that if cardiovascular disease has a hereditary component then their children and other family members would also experience cardiovascular disease. Some people can do their best to live a healthy lifestyle but still experience cardiovascular disease because of their family history. But like Buchanan, people can try to adhere to a healthy lifestyle to offset their family history of cardiovascular disease.

Conditions that contribute to cardiovascular disease, like obesity, also have a hereditary component. Therefore, higher rates of these conditions among Black people may at least partially explain their higher rates of cardiovascular disease. But these conditions also have a social component. For instance, proximity to grocery stores with healthy foods, culturally defined eating habits, experiences with racism, and racism-related stress can all contribute to obesity. Similarly, Black families with a history of cardiovascular disease often have shared living environments and thus experience the same factors that contribute to cardiovascular disease.[30]

Slavery Hypertension Hypothesis

Although cardiovascular disease has a hereditary component, there is a common and persistent myth that Black people are predisposed to hypertension (which contributes to cardiovascular disease) as an evolutionary trait inherited from our enslaved African ancestors. According to the theory, the conditions on the slave ships that were used to force Africans to the Americas during the Middle Passage were inhumane, filthy, and violent, and they were not given proper nutrition or hydration. This made surviving the journey difficult, and in fact many of the enslaved Africans did not survive these harsh conditions. The Africans who did survive, however, were those whose bodies retained more salt. The idea was that since Africans were subjected to heat, limited water, and salt while in Africa, they developed a predisposition to salt retention. In fact, White people would often lick the faces of Africans they wanted to enslave. They believed a lick to the skin could test the amount of salt in their body and that Africans with less salty skin would die during the journey to the Americas, while Africans with saltier skin would survive long enough to be enslaved.[31] The belief is then that modern African Americans inherited a salt retention gene from our enslaved African ancestors and that is the cause of our higher rates of hypertension. Sometimes this is called the "slavery hypertension hypothesis."

This theory is very prevalent in popular culture. Even journalist and TV personality Oprah Winfrey repeated this theory on a 2007 episode of her talk show *Oprah* and TV personality Dr. Oz supported the theory. This theory is also frequently taught in medical schools as an explanation for differences in Black people and White people's rates of hypertension. The American Heart Association and the popular WebMD website both state that Black people's higher rates of hypertension may stem from their African ancestry. Even the CDC has stated that Black people's sensitivity to salt and their resulting greater risk of hypertension has a genetic explanation. The slavery hypertension hypothesis, though, is comprised of half-truths and half-falsehoods.

Although there may be some hereditary component to hypertension, the slavery hypertension hypothesis is a myth not supported with proper research or any credible data. In fact, most of the sources on this theory are not peer-reviewed and stem from abstracts or conference reports. Much of the current and credible research has shown this theory to be implausible. For example, researchers found that salt-resistant subjects and salt-sensitive subjects retain the same amount of sodium. This means that salt retention is unimportant to distinguishing salt-sensitive and salt-resistant subjects. In fact, other research tells us that differences in salt sensitivity between Black and White individuals is not significant.

It is possible that one day we will have definitive scientific evidence for Black people's heritable predisposition for hypertension. This evidence, however, would have to be tied to ethnicity and ancestry, not race. And heritability would likely prove to only be but one of many factors that influences their higher rates of hypertension. But until this happens, racial myths should not serve as a placeholder for what we do not know. The slavery hypertension hypothesis is another example of scientific racism in which racism, and the idea that Black people are genetically and evolutionary inferior, is used to explain meaningful, but largely social differences between the races. The problem is that scientific racism has been continuously discredited by rigorous research. Yet scientific explanations for poor health outcomes for Black people tend to be used as a replacement for more meritorious social explanations. Resigning to scientific racism instead of social causes also discourages solutions that can address the problem such as policy changes, medical intervention, and public health campaigns. The slavery hypertension myth is another instance of pathologizing Black people and not pathologizing the environments in which Black people live.

Social Risk Factors: Where We Live

Where we live is a great predictor of our health. The neighborhoods where we live often determine our proximity to crime, recreation, stable schools, healthy food, and noise and light pollution. All of these neighborhood characteristics can influence the prevalence of cardiovascular disease. For example, between 2002 and 2009 researchers studied over 27,000 adults, most of whom were Black, female, and had low incomes. At the start of the study none of the participants had cardiovascular disease; cardiovascular disease, however, among other things, was one of the outcomes tracked by researchers. Most of the participants lived in low-income, disadvantaged neighborhoods. After five years the researchers found that 16 percent of the participants developed cardiovascular disease and the worse their neighborhood was the more increase in heart failure among the participants they found. Some of the participants that lived in the poorest neighborhoods had a 24 percent greater risk of developing cardiovascular disease compared to the participants that lived in somewhat better neighborhoods.[32] It is worth noting that the neighborhoods themselves did not cause their cardiovascular disease rather the associated characteristics of the neighborhoods and the social lives of the people who live in these neighborhoods likely did.

Poorer neighborhoods can also explain differences in Black people's experiences with cardiovascular disease as compared to White people's experiences with cardiovascular disease since Black people are more likely to live in poorer neighborhoods.[33] For instance, as further discussed in chapter 4, poorer neighborhoods often lack the social determinants of sleep health like low to no noise pollution or little to no air pollution, access to recreation, and feelings of safety and security. Black people are more likely to live in poorer neighborhoods which correlates with their higher rates of sleeplessness when compared to White people. Higher rates of sleeplessness have been linked to higher rates of hypertension, which also disproportionately affects Black people.[34] Sleeplessness is just one of the pathways to poor cardiovascular health created by our social lives.

Racial Discrimination

Racial discrimination is disproportionately experienced by people of color. Being on the receiving end of racial discrimination is also bad for people's health. At least one pathway for racial discrimination to cause harm is the stress it causes, the biological processes it disrupts, and the physiological ways our bodies react to stress. One manifestation of the stress of racial discrimination is cardiovascular disease. The stress of racial discrimination has been linked to Black people's higher risk of cardiovascular disease.[35] The stress itself can harm their heart health but it can also increase Black people's propensity to engage in unhealthy behaviors that increase their risks of cardiovascular disease. Stress induced by racial discrimination can also make it harder to manage previously diagnosed cardiovascular disease.

Racial discrimination in clinical care also impacts Black people's cardiovascular health. When seeking health care for cardiovascular disease, Black people's symptoms of cardiovascular disease are often not taken seriously by clinicians. As a result, sometimes life-saving cardiac care is either withheld or delivered when it is too late to be of any benefit. For example, in a study of over 17,000 heart attack patients hospitalized in four US states between 2000 and 2014, researchers found that Black people were less likely than White people to receive common medications for cardiovascular disease even when they should have been given medication under standard treatment guidelines. Black people are also less likely than White people to receive more aggressive medical interventions like bypass surgery or angioplasty.[36] Other studies suggest that Black people, among other people of color, experience racial inequities in receiving cardiovascular treatments such as cardiac catheterization and surgical revascularization.[37] But many cardiologists, however, do not see their role or their institution's role in racial disparities in cardiovascular disease and are generally unaware of the social causes of racial disparities in cardiovascular disease.[38] Instead, they blame patients' unhealthy behaviors or their access to health insurance, showing a lack of understanding of racial disparities in health care and how those racial disparities function within Black people's lives.

How health care providers view Black patients with symptoms of cardiovascular disease matters because speed is a necessity for cardiovascular care. How quickly people can access health care can mean the difference between surviving a cardiovascular event such as a stroke or heart attack and disability or death. One study, however, found that despite quality improvement initiatives, for Black people, it is less likely that the time they enter a health care facility to the time they are treated for a cardiac event will be under ninety minutes, which does not meet the typical standard for good cardiac care.[39] The study also found that Black people had longer revascularization times than White people. Overall, the delays in treatment were longer for Black men than other racial and gender groups. When providers' racial biases make it so there is an increase in time before they are seen by physicians, then it is the very nature of health care that stands in the way of Black people receiving the cardiovascular care they need to survive.

Providers' racial biases also contribute to racial disparities in cardiovascular disease by discouraging Black people from seeing a physician when it is necessary. Either from their own experiences or from the experiences of family and friends, Black people are aware of racial biases in health care. They know that health care providers can exhibit racist attitudes toward Black people and that those racist attitudes can contribute to racist behaviors that affect their health. Narratives about health care experiences shared within Black communities are powerful, influential, and long-lasting. Black people's experiences with racism in health care run deep, plus they are consistently reinforced with new experiences of racism.

Calvin and colleagues sum up how racism affects Black people's rates of cardiovascular disease with a review of three levels of racism—(1) institutional racism, (2) personally mediated racism, and (3) internalized racism.[40] First, institutionalized racism in the form of racist policies that result in inferior education, under-resourced neighborhoods, and lesser access to employment and income influence Black people's socioeconomic status (SES). And whether measured by our neighborhood, education, or wealth, SES directly correlates with our cardiovascular health. Namely, the lower a person's SES, the greater their risk for cardiovascular disease. And as we know, SES maps onto race with Black people and other marginalized groups consistently having lower SES.

Second, personally mediated racism or the individual experience of racial discrimination also affects Black people's experience of cardiovascular disease. Sometimes racism is called *perceived racism,* indicating that racism is in the eye of the beholder. Like many other scholars I do not use the term *perceived racism* because the term necessarily casts doubt on whether a person experienced racism, making their experiences a matter of truthhood or falsehood. But whether a person *actually* experienced racism is unimportant (as if we could objectively determine it); whether a person experienced racism or not, the effects of racism on their health is the same. Additionally, questioning the validity of a Black person's claim of racism is to commit violence against them; it's another instance of not believing Black people's experiences. Black people have spent a lifetime in a Black body and that gives them better knowledge of when they have experienced racism than any other person. What matters is that racism causes race-related stress and stress contributes to cardiovascular disease. Personally mediated racism is an environmental stimulus that triggers psychological and physiological responses in our bodies, similar to the "fight or flight" response. Stress activates our immune, neuroendocrine, and cardiovascular systems. Similarly, we may experience denial, anger, hopelessness, or fear after experiencing racism, which all can contribute to bodily stressors.

Lastly, internalized racism, or when we believe negative stereotypes about our own racial group that are perpetuated by dominant racial groups, can also affect Black people's health. Calvin and colleagues note that Black people can internalize the blatant and subtle racist stereotypes that can be seen be seen in everyday American culture.[41] Film, TV, social media, all can portray Black people using negative stereotypes that harm Black people's sense of identity and self-worth, and undermine their very existence. Stereotypical depictions of Black people can create a stigma of Black inferiority, which can influence the ways that Black patients are treated by health care providers. These negative depictions of Black people and the internalized racism they create can also encourage negative emotions. The distress of negative emotions is a possible pathway through which internalized racism contributes to Black people's risk of cardiovascular disease.

Although social, cultural, and political determinants of health such as the quality of our neighborhoods, access to income, education, and health care, and our experiences with different kinds of racial discrimination affect all Black people, there are some instances when these social determinants of health affect people of different genders in different ways. Black women and Black men have different experiences with cardiovascular disease. Their sometimes differing experiences with the social determinants of health may be one explanation for this. It is important to note that the research on Black men and women's cardiovascular health does rely on only two genders. Because this is how the available research uses gender, I too will focus on men and women. The following section, however, is by no means an endorsement of the view that there are only two genders nor an endorsement that "men" does not include transgender men, and similarly that "women" does not include transgender women.

Black Women

At her annual checkup Tasha Benjamin's physician looked at her electrocardiogram readings and told her that she had experienced a heart attack. Benjamin, a thirty-six-year-old Black woman, thought he was joking and told him "Well, I do have a husband and 4 kids."[42] She thought the physician was joking because she was unaware of any heart attack nor did she experience any symptoms of a heart attack. Benjamin had a "silent" heart attack. The heart attack had temporarily blocked blood flow to a part of her heart, damaging the heart muscle. A year before, however, she was diagnosed with high blood pressure. With a change in her diet and daily medication, though, she was able to improve her blood pressure readings and stop taking medication. Seven years after finding out she had a "silent" heart attack, Benjamin's heart is in good condition. Reflecting on her heart attack, she believes that the stress of being married to an active-duty marine who was often deployed, leaving her to care for their four children by herself, while also worrying about her husband's safety, may have contributed to her heart attack.

Cardiovascular disease greatly affects all Americans. But for Black women like Benjamin, cardiovascular disease is slightly more deadly. Black women are one of the groups most affected by cardiovascular disease, including being at risk for earlier onset of cardiovascular disease. Of all Black women over the age of twenty, about half have had some kind of cardiovascular disease.[43] A 2019 study found that Black women aged eighteen to thirty-five had a 58 percent higher likelihood of developing hypertension compared to White women.[44] Black women also have a higher risk of stroke and at an earlier age compared to White people of any gender and Black men.[45] Black women are also slightly more likely to die from cardiovascular disease than White women.[46] Reading stories like Benjamin's and other Black women, one common factor seems to be stress, particularly among Black women with many domestic responsibilities and Black women with professional, high-functioning careers.

Cherée Johnson, a Black woman, petite in stature, still at her college weight, made time to exercise and maintain a healthy diet while performing her duties as an international corporate lawyer.[47] Johnson also has a husband and two young children. After having a sharp pain in her chest for about a year, she went to see a physician who told her that she was just stressed. Her blood tests and chest X-ray were also normal. But in 2018, the day before a big presentation, she collapsed on her way to the bathroom in the middle of the night. Before going to the hospital Johnson got dressed for work, grabbed her laptop and phone thinking she could do her presentation after she was done at the hospital. Once there, however, to her disbelief, she was informed that she was having a heart attack. Physicians inserted a stent restoring blood flow after finding a blocked artery in her heart. The physician told her that the artery was 99 percent blocked and that she had been having a heart attack for eighteen hours. Eventually returning to work, Johnson had a new mindset:

The heart attack forced me to stop and prioritize what was important in my life. That meant my health and my family. I now approach work with much more confidence and courage than stress and fear." Johnson worried, that as an executive, people may see her as weak after having a heart attack, but instead decided that it was more important to be courageous and resilient.

Like Tasha Benjamin, Cherée Johnson also seemed to have a high functioning, likely stressful (at least in part) life, including a demanding career. Vanessa Taylor, another career-driven Black woman with cardiovascular disease also believes stress contributed to her poor health.[48] Like many other Black women she believed that she had to work harder than her peers to succeed:

When I was younger, I was very career driven. I had to work harder because I was a Black woman in a predominantly White organization. I wasn't allowing myself time to decompress and effectively manage my stress.

Stress affects everyone's health, regardless of race or gender, but Black women have gender- and race-specific stressors. It is common for Black women to fulfill the role of family matriarch and facilitate the emotional and financial wellbeing of family members as well as caregiving duties. Black women also work outside the home more than White and Latinx women.[49] To properly address Black women's experiences with cardiovascular disease, we have to explore their unique stressors and address how those stressors impact their health in ways that it does not impact other people's health.

Black women's experiences of cardiovascular disease also differ from others' experiences because women exhibit symptoms differently than men.[50] Women's symptoms tend to be more subtle like fatigue or nausea, which they may attribute to being tired or overworked. Women can also have a heart attack but never experience chest pains and instead experience shortness of breath or lightheadedness. Physicians may attribute these symptoms to something other than cardiovascular disease, especially in young women. This is one of the reasons why health care providers' biases matter; their biases can lead them to ignore Black women's symptoms of cardiovascular disease and dismiss their complaints of poor health. Biases can also lead them to give Black women lesser quality care. For instance, when we look at the intersection of race and gender, physicians are significantly less likely to recommend catheterization for cardiac events for Black women when compared to White men.[51] Relatedly, it is important for providers to be knowledgeable about how cardiovascular disease presents in women and the rates of cardiovascular disease in younger Black women so they can provide proper care and not continue to contribute to racial and gender disparities in cardiovascular disease.

Black Men

Highlighting racial biases in cardiac care, Dr. Kimberly Manning tells the story of her father, a Black man seeking treatment for what turned out to be an acute myocardial infarction:[52]

> My father called me when I was a senior resident. I was in the CCU on my final rotation, and we were chatting on the phone and dad told me that he was having shoulder pain. He was an avid golfer at the time and had played a few holes of golf, but it was a very unusual way he was describing this pain. He saw his primary care doctor, who gave him some Motrin, and he called the doctor back and said, "This is really not right. This is not normal. Something's wrong." And the doctor sort of trivialized his feelings and said, "You know, you played 36 holes of golf in a tournament—of course your shoulder's going to hurt." But my dad had risk factors. He had a family history of coronary disease. He was hypertensive. He had hyperlipidemia. He was in care, but still, he had risk factors, and finally, as we were chatting, he told me that his pain felt like biting ice with his tooth. I was like, "That sounds visceral, Dad." I knew it didn't sound like musculoskeletal pain from swinging a golf club.

Despite his obvious symptoms of acute myocardial infarction, after ten to twelve hours Manning's father was not offered cardiac catheterization. Knowing how biases affect health care and existing racial disparities in health care, Manning coached her father on what to say so that he would get the care that he needed:

> And you know, because I know how powerful bias is, I essentially told him to go to the hospital, and I told him to lie. I told him when he got there to say he had chest pain, that he was diaphoretic, that he had dyspnea on exertion—none of which he had. All he had was severe shoulder pain, but I thought that it sounded cardiac, and that is what got him through triage.

With his daughter's assistance, Manning's father was able to work around the health care system to get admitted to the hospital. Manning knew that Black people often have worse health outcomes when compared to White people and she didn't want her father to fall victim to racial disparities in health outcomes we so often see:

> And the reason I say it's an equity issue is because what I know for sure is that if my dad had not . . . if he had come into the triage and just kind of said what he said [to me], we know that there is plenty of data that supports if you have four people—a Black man, a Black woman, a White man, a White woman—all with the exact same story, they will often have different outcomes.

Black men like Manning's father have two barriers to proper cardiovascular health: (1) racial disparities in the social determinants of health that influence their disproportionate rates of cardiovascular disease, and (2) access to proper health care.

Black men are disproportionately affected by cardiovascular disease. Among all Black adult men, 60 percent have cardiovascular disease.[53] In some instances, like with hypertension, Black men are more likely to have a higher incidence of cardiovascular disease than White or Latinx men. Like the celebrity film director, John Singleton, Black men also have the highest increase in death from hypertension.[54] Overall, Black men have slightly more deaths from cardiovascular disease than Black women at 54,000 and 52,000 respectively, per year. Black men also have slightly more instances of coronary cardiovascular disease, including deaths from the disease, and heart attacks than Black women. And even though they have similar risks of cardiovascular disease as White men, Black men are twice as likely as White men to die from cardiovascular events like heart attack.[55] In general, when we compare Black men's experiences with cardiovascular disease to other populations, we see that Black men continue to have some of the worst cardiovascular health outcomes.

While some other populations' risk for cardiovascular disease has fallen over the years, Black men's risk has increased. For example, a 2018 study found that between 2011 and 2014, 65 percent of Black men between the ages of forty and seventy-nine were considered high risk for having a heart attack and stroke within the next ten years. Their risk, however, just a decade earlier was 54 percent. White men's risk of cardiovascular disease, on the other hand only increased to 48 percent. Black women and White women, in the same age group, risk of cardiovascular disease fell from 15 percent to 11 percent and 10 percent to 5 percent, respectively. Based on this study, the researchers concluded that Black men are a high-risk group for cardiovascular disease, making them a vulnerable population.[56] When calling a group a "vulnerable population," however, we have to question what makes them vulnerable.

Black men's cardiovascular health is jeopardized by their general low likelihood of undergoing routine health examinations. One study suggested that addressing medical mistrust and concerns about masculinity and vulnerability would improve their rates of routine health examinations.[57] Increasing their interaction with health care providers would then likely better their cardiovascular health. For example, more interaction with health care providers could help decrease rates of diabetes. Fourteen percent of Black men have been diagnosed with diabetes, and 31.9 percent have prediabetes. More interaction with health care providers could mean early detection and treatment for diabetes before it becomes a contributing factor to their rates of cardiovascular disease. But this study's recommendations highlight that mistrust and cultural norms are at least some of the barriers that stand in the way of Black men's access to health care. Relying on interventions that repair the trust between Black people and health care and campaigns that target the specific needs of Black men would help them have more access to health care. But this is a burden that health care must take on, as the perpetrator of mistrust. Black men did not break the relationship and are therefore not responsible for fixing it.

There are other social barriers that stand in the way of Black men's cardiovascular health. A lack of adequate income is a barrier to health that many people face, but for Black men the barrier is even more pronounced given their generally lower incomes. Although Black men's incomes are slightly more than Black women, neither group has managed to close income gaps that exist between Black and White and Asian people. Black men's average income is about $42,000, while White men's income is about $60,000.[58] One study found that even when Black men are employed in corporate type jobs they still make less money than White men in the same positions. Black men are the only group that never reach pay parity with White men when we examine average income.[59] As of 2021, Black men also have the lowest rate of employment compared to all racial and gender groups.[60] Black men's employment rates, however, have to be understood in relation to their high incarceration rates. Although incarceration rates are dropping, Black men are still significantly more likely to be incarcerated than White and Latinx men, which affects how many Black men are employed in America.[61]

Black men's lower rates of employment and income are pathways for cardiovascular disease given employment's relationship to our experiences with stress. Black people in general report higher levels of stress (along with Latinx and Asian people) than White people. But among Black people, those with lower incomes report experiencing more stressful life events and those events causing greater distress than White people.[62] For Black men, lesser income and employment can mean higher rates of stress. For instance, when people do not have the money to buy life's necessities like food and housing for themselves and their families as well as those things we would consider luxuries, it can cause people to stress. Additionally, societal and cultural norms may encourage Black men to see themselves as their family's breadwinner and attach their value to how much money they bring to their families, causing more employment related stress. One way for health care providers to help Black men lower their risk of cardiovascular disease is to be aware of the cultural, racial, and gender norms that are a part of Black men's lives.[63]

Black men's cardiovascular health is also influenced by their rates of poor mental health and experiences with depression and anxiety, which can be brought on by stressful life events.[64] One study found that after Latinx people, Black people have the highest rates of depression. The researchers concluded that one of the reasons for their experiences with depression was a lack of employment and lack of health insurance coverage (which is often tied to employment).[65] The researchers also stressed the importance of access to mental health care for at-risk groups, which is hindered by a lack of health insurance. Black men's lesser contact with primary care physicians can also affect their access to mental health care. And again, societal, cultural, gender, and racial norms may discourage Black men from seeking the mental health care they need, associating it with weakness or other negative emotions, if they can even afford care.[66]

Racially Concordant Care and Other Solutions

There are some systemic policies and actions that health care institutions and public health organizations can take to better Black people's cardiac health. One action that has gained some support, as well as criticism, is racially concordant care, sometimes called race-matching. Race-matching is when a physician of a certain race is intentionally assigned to care for a patient of the same race. For some racial minority patients, race-matching has proved to facilitate better health outcomes. For instance, studies have found that race-matching improves patient trust,[67] consent to preventative care like screenings for diseases,[68] and a likelihood of following cardiovascular disease treatment recommendations.[69] Race-matching has also shown to decrease racial biases' role in patient care.[70]

There have been specific studies that found race-matching could reduce Black people's experiences with cardiovascular disease. A 2018 study of 1,300 Black men in Oakland, California found that when Black men were seen by Black physicians, they were more likely to consent to free preventative measures like diabetes and cholesterol screenings than when they were seen by non-Black physicians.[71] Researchers suggest that race matching could reduce the Black-White mortality gap caused by cardiovascular disease by sixteen deaths per 100,000 per year, which is 19 percent of the gap,[72] highlighting the need for more Black physicians.

The benefits of race-matching in health care may be underscored by how few Black physicians exist. As of 2018, Black people made up about 5 percent of all physicians in the United States.[73] This means that every Black person who wants a Black physician cannot feasibly have one. This also highlights the burden that Black physicians who are practicing may feel trying to meet the demand of Black patients. It may not be fair to ask Black physicians, who already experience racism and other forms of discrimination in their own profession from colleagues and patients, to also take on the burden of fixing health care's racism problem. Assigning Black physicians to Black patients also may discourage non-Black physicians from addressing their anti-Black racial biases and working to give better care to Black patients.[74]

Another way to address Black people's cardiac health is to address structural racism. In fact, the American Heart Association (AHA) has named structural racism as a driver of racial disparities in cardiovascular disease.[75] As a part of a presidential advisory, the AHA revealed that their review of structural racism in America and the current state of cardiovascular disease revealed that "racism persists; racism is experienced; and the task of dismantling racism must belong to all of society. It cannot be accomplished by affected individuals alone." Additionally, in their review they named social determinants as a target for reforming cardiovascular disease among marginalized racial groups:

The path forward requires our commitment to transforming the conditions of historically marginalized communities, improving the quality of housing and neighborhood environments of these populations, advocating for policies that eliminate inequities in access to economic opportunities, quality education, and health care, and enhancing allyship among racial and ethnic groups.

The AHA statement highlights that the causes of racial disparities in cardiovascular disease are not individual, and therefore, the solutions should not be individual changes alone. Instead, we have to address the systemic forces behind Black people's poor cardiac health. This includes advancing research on the joint effects of different types of racism (structural, interpersonal, and anti-Black racism). Similarly, other researchers have also drawn attention to a need for an examination of the social determinants of health and an intersectional understanding of the people most at risk for cardiovascular disease, like Black people.[76]

Conclusion

There are many issues related to Black people's experiences with cardiovascular disease that I did not discuss. For instance, aligning with race-based medicine, some physicians prescribe certain drugs to Black people based on the belief that those drugs work better for African Americans. For instance, the drug Bidil, has been specifically used to treat heart failure in self-identified African Americans. It has a long and complicated history with health care providers, researchers, and scholars who want Black people to have better health, but find race-based medicine, like Bidil, at best questionable, at worst, scientifically incorrect.[77] Bidil represents an approach to correcting Black people's experiences with cardiovascular disease that focuses on treating the disease after Black people have it. This chapter, however, examines the social and cultural determinants of Black people's experiences so that their rates of cardiovascular disease can be prevented. Remedying Black people's experiences with low incomes, poverty, and racism, including racial discrimination in health care, can all help Black people have lower rates of cardiovascular disease. Additionally, targeting their experiences with diseases that contribute to cardiovascular disease, such as diabetes, can also lower their risk of cardiovascular disease.

Exploring the social and cultural determinants of Black people's rates of cardiovascular disease adds a new dimension to how being Black intersects with health in America and how we treat Black people with poor health. It is easier to moralize Black people's health; it is easier to say that Black people have poor health because of their bad actions. When we do, however, health care and public health agencies do not have to respond to structural racism's effects on Black people's health, including the ways they have contributed. If we moralize Black people's health then we do not have to acknowledge the interconnectedness of social systems and their oppressive behaviors and Black people's health outcomes. But when we explore Black people's experiences with cardiovascular disease, for instance, we see that although cardiovascular disease is deadly and disabling for all people, the lived experience of being Black adds a unique layer of vulnerability and burden. Living as a Black person means living with racism in everyday life, even when seeking health care. This is something White people do not experience, and therefore it is not a threat to their cardiovascular health. Cardiovascular disease is just one example of how Black people's identities function within our society to contribute to their rates of disease, while they live with the social, personal, and financial costs.

Discussion Questions

1. What are other social determinants of Black people's rates of cardiovascular disease?

2. What policies could health care institutions and public health organizations create to help Black people have less cardiovascular disease?

3. How do we acknowledge systemic racism's effect on Black people's rates of cardiovascular disease and also hold Black people accountable for their choices that affect their health?

4. Do you think race-matching is a worthwhile health care practice? What are some benefits and drawbacks for clinicians and patients?

5. What are the types of targeted health campaigns that could change Black people's experiences with cardiovascular disease?

4

Does Where We Sleep Matter?

Kimberly Turner is a 55-year-old African American woman living in Brooklyn, New York.[1] Turner was having some strange experiences. The people around her would suddenly disappear. While driving, she would stop at a red light and then before she knew it, cars would honk their horn at her, signaling the light had turned green. She was essentially losing time. Turner didn't realize that she was falling asleep during the day and doing so at inopportune times. She was tired all the time. And when she did sleep, she would wake up with headaches. One day Turner's husband told her that while sleeping she had stopped breathing. At first, she didn't believe him because she had no knowledge of this happening to her.

Her physician recommended she complete a sleep study where she would go to a facility and sleep overnight while being monitored by medical equipment and staff. Two minutes into her study, however, the whole thing had to be stopped because Turner stopped breathing too many times. She was eventually diagnosed with sleep apnea and was told to wear a CPAP (continuous positive airway pressure) mask while she slept at night to keep her airways open. After using the CPAP mask, her headaches were gone and she was more alert during the day.

Sleep is vital to our biological, physical, mental, and emotional health. Sleep allows our body to reset and restore itself at the most basic cellular and physiological level.[2] Poor sleep, however, makes it hard for our brain to function, complicating all activities of life from the most basic to the most complex. When we have not slept well, it becomes extremely difficult to pursue hobbies, careers,

Black Health. Keisha Ray, Oxford University Press. © Oxford University Press 2023.
DOI: 10.1093/oso/9780197620267.003.0005

familial duties, and maintain relationships with other people. Poor sleep can also contribute to diseases and illnesses such as hypertension and diabetes. At the public health level, sleeplessness can cause motor vehicle crashes and errors while working at our jobs. Our sleeplessness can cause harm to ourselves, but also to the people around us. This is likely why the Centers for Disease Control and Prevention (CDC) has declared sleeplessness a public health issue.[3] This declaration signals just how important sleep is to individuals and to a healthy society. Therefore, who sleeps, who does not sleep, and the individual and collective health problems sleeplessness creates are a necessary part of any conversation on health. And like many other health outcomes among Americans, sleeplessness falls along racial lines.

Data provided by scholars in disciplines like public health, biomedical sciences, psychology, and sociology show that there are racial disparities in quality and quantity of sleep between the different races.[4] Specifically, in America, Black people sleep less and have lesser quality of sleep than White people. Some studies have found that Black people spend about 15 percent of the night in deep sleep, or the phase of our sleep cycle that is the most restorative, while White people spend about 23 percent of the night in deep sleep. In general, Black people spend more time in light sleep while White people spend more time in deep sleep.[5] Using data from wrist actigraphy and sleep logs, some researchers found that Black men get the least amount of sleep in a night (5.1 hours), followed by Black women (5.9 hours) and White men (6.1 hours). Of all the racial and gender groups studied, White women slept the most amount of time (6.7 hours).[6]

Racial disparities in sleep are concerning in their own right because when sleeplessness falls along racial lines, the rejuvenating benefits of sleep will also fall along racial lines. But racial disparities in sleep are also concerning because some researchers believe they may map onto racial disparities observed in health outcomes like diabetes, heart disease, mortality, and other health outcomes.[7] For example, Black men get the least amount of sleep and they have the lowest life expectancy of all racial and gender groups.[8] Is there a connection between these two health outcomes? Perhaps, but it is certainly worthy of investigation. This also leads to the more general question, "Have high rates of disease contributed to Black people getting less sleep or has getting less sleep contributed to higher rates of diseases in the Black population?" The simple and not so simple answer is, likely yes. The relationship between health and sleep is co-dependent—poor health causes poor sleep and poor sleep causes poor health. When we examine the sociocultural context of sleep, however, we do find that sleeplessness among Black people is more likely influenced by lesser access to social determinants of health (income, employment, healthy environment, etc.), than naturally occurring higher rates of disease. Given that many of the social determinants of health are also the social determinants of sleep, and we know that Black people experience inequities in the former, there is indication that sleeplessness is not inherent to being Black.

In this chapter I discuss the social, cultural, and political factors that influence Black people's higher rates of sleeplessness. This includes housing injustices that have kept Black people in resourced deprived neighborhoods, environmental injustices that expose Black people to toxins, and racial discrimination that forces Black people to be watchful for race based harm. I also discuss how health care and public health's advocacy for sleep hygiene, or tips for better sleep, contribute to our misunderstanding of racial disparities in sleep. Cultural practices like later bedtimes also play a role in Black people's sleep quality. Examining these pathways of sleeplessness ultimately demonstrates how Black people's health is endangered when they do not have access to the social determinants of health.

Housing

How well we sleep is tied to where we live, and presumably sleep. How well we sleep is also tied to with whom we live and sleep near and how safe and supported we feel in our homes and communities. But where we live is socially, culturally, and politically influenced and often tied to the social effects of race, class, and gender. As such it is no surprise that Black people sleep less than White people since the socio-political institutions that influence sleep, such as housing, have been historically oppressive and discriminatory toward Black people.

In general, Black people are more likely than White people to live in poorer neighborhoods, even when their income would firmly put them in the middle class.[9] Poorer neighborhoods, or neighborhoods that are often intentionally economically and resource deprived by social and political forces outside of inhabitants' control, tend to have features that are not conducive to proper sleep quality. Poorer neighborhoods are often characterized by noise pollutants, such as noise from neighbors, vehicles on the highway, sirens from emergency vehicles, or noise from local businesses, and they all interrupt sleep. Poorer neighborhoods can have other characteristics that undermine sleep like excessive artificial light (e.g., street lamps), and inadequate heating and cooling (either because the home does not have the proper equipment or because the residents cannot afford to properly heat and cool their home).[10] Since poorer neighborhoods are disproportionately populated by people of color, they are disproportionately exposed to these kinds of sleep deterrents.[11]

People who live in less affluent neighborhoods may also have a heightened sense of vigilance, or alertness due to fears about their own and/or their family's safety.[12] When we feel safe and do not have to worry about our own or our family's safety, we sleep better. As Lucy Hale, the editor of the journal *Sleep Health* says, "If you know somebody in your neighborhood who has had a break-in, you might feel pretty uncomfortable shutting your eyes falling asleep while your two or three children are sleeping in the room next door and no one else is there to protect them."[13] Hypervigilance is a matter of feeling unprotected and insecure in our own home and prevents the mind from being at ease, which is needed for proper sleep.

Housing is a major determinant of sleep health. Noise pollutants, artificial light, hypervigilance, and feelings of not being safe are all a part of what makes a home an unsuitable place for sleep. And it is not an accident that many Black people live in poorer neighborhoods that have these characteristics. Rather, where Black people live and sleep is often the result of intentional and strategically implemented discriminatory housing laws. If poor housing is a pathway to poor sleep, then housing laws, both historic and contemporary, act as structural barriers to Black people's proper sleep health.

Where We Sleep

Black people choosing to live in economically poor neighborhoods and White people choosing to live in wealthy neighborhoods is a myth the US Supreme Court once tried to use to justify segregated neighborhoods with differing access to resources. Instead, in *The Color of Law*, Richard Rothstein argues that racial segregation in housing was intentionally created by our local, state, and federal governments.[14] For example, Rothstein states that, in response to a shortage of homes for Americans, in 1933 the US government gave homes to middle- to lower-class White families. Black families, on the other hand, were put in large urban projects. Additionally, the Federal Housing Administration (FHA) made it difficult for Black people to buy homes and move out of urban projects by refusing to insure mortgages in "Black neighborhoods." The FHA did, however, subsidize home builders who developed "White neighborhoods" and did not sell homes in "White neighborhoods" to Black people. Policies such as these were meant to keep Black people from living in White, affluent neighborhoods that were safe and near affluent public schools. Instead, as White neighborhoods were thriving with government assistance, Black neighborhoods were neglected and continued to deteriorate while receiving little to no government assistance. Government at all levels withheld the resources and money that Black neighborhoods needed to provide their residents with safe, healthy, and prosperous lives.

Although illegal, discriminatory housing practices are still used to keep neighborhoods racially segregated—now they are just less overt, and more underhanded, making it harder to be revealed. Exclusionary zoning, which dates back to the 1910s, is sometimes called "snob zoning."[15] Although made illegal in 1917,[16] exclusionary zoning laws are meant to work around anti-discriminatory housing laws. They rely on existing and newly created zoning laws to prohibit companies from building certain types of housing structures like apartment buildings, multi-family homes, or homes with lesser square footage in typically affluent neighborhoods. Although many people who support these laws say that they are engaging in "rational land-use planning" and are protecting the value of their homes,[17] the results of these laws are undeniable—they keep Black people, other people of color, and poor people out of supposed "White neighborhoods." Exclusionary zoning is still so relevant to where Black people live that the United States White House website made it a topic of discussion on their blog in 2021. The White House blog named exclusionary zoning as a priority for the President Biden administration in its effort to decrease social inequities.[18] Exclusionary zoning is an act of institutional racism that keeps Black people from accessing homes in safe, affluent, and properly resourced neighborhoods. As such, exclusionary zoning becomes a means of withholding proper health, and proper sleep, from Black people.

Where Black people live, thus where Black people sleep, is rooted in discriminatory housing policies. Segregate housing policies like redlining, where banks would draw a red line on a map to indicate where banks would not offer housing loans because they were considered "Black neighborhoods," have had lasting effects on where Black people live and sleep. The federal Fair Housing Act of 1968, as a part of the Civil Rights Act of 1968, was enacted as a response to widespread discrimination in housing. It prohibits discrimination in housing based on nationality, sex, religion, national origin, sex, and race.[19] Despite the Fair Housing Act, some White people and wealthy people found ways to manipulate existing laws to keep Black people and poor people in "Black neighborhoods" and out of "White neighborhoods." Even after the Fair Housing Act made it legal for Black people to buy homes in "White neighborhoods," Black people could no longer afford to buy homes in these neighborhoods.[20] If they had been allowed to buy homes in these neighborhoods when White people were receiving government assistance to purchase homes, however, then they could have afforded the homes. By the time Black people were allowed to purchase homes in these more affluent neighborhoods, they were priced out. Being priced out of home ownership, Rothstein argues, also prevented Black people from capitalizing on the wealth and social mobility that home equity provides to homeowners. He argues that White parents used the equity in their homes to send their children to college, giving them a head start in life. Their children were also able to care for their aging parents and aging parents did not have to rely on their children to care for them as they aged. Parents were also able to leave their children money after their death, once again helping to secure their children's future. This is an example of how institutional racism affects generations of Black families— White families had help from the US government to build generational wealth, while generational wealth and its benefits were withheld from Black people.

In instances when the government did intervene on the behalf of Black people who wanted to purchase homes, it often created programs that made them easy prey for predatory companies.[21] For example, in the 1960s and 1970s the government enacted low-income homeownership programs meant to help Black people purchase homes, in particular the large population of poor- to middle-class Black women, who were often the head of their households. Black women, often viewed home ownership as central to the American dream and wanting their own piece of the American dream, were open to taking on these mortgages. Mortgage lenders, however, viewed these women as vulnerable homeowners likely to fail to pay their mortgage and have their homes foreclosed upon. And since the terms of the newly enacted government sponsored programs ensured lenders that they would be paid in full for any house that fell into foreclosure, lenders were incentivized to put Black women into homes that they could not afford. These programs made Black women easy targets for real estate and mortgage bankers to take advantage of their desire to own property and give them mortgages that based on their income, they knew the women could not afford.

Home ownership and its financial benefits are still elusive for many Black people. The gap between Black and White home ownership continues to widen to levels not seen since the 1960s.[22] While about 70 percent of White people owned homes in 2017, home ownership among Black people was about 45 percent. When it comes to Black and White millennials, homeownership rates are similarly disproportionate with about 13 percent of Black millennials owning homes and about 37 percent of White millennials owning homes. At least one contributing systemic factor to this gap in home ownership is racism in money lending for home ownership. In 2019 researchers found that home lenders were less likely to give home loans to Black people than they were to White people even when their financial backgrounds, such as credit scores, were identical.[23] Researchers believe there to be racial bias in the algorithms major home lenders use to determine who qualifies for a home loan.

The story behind how Black people came to live in poorer neighborhoods includes policies that supported White supremacy and Black inferiority. The idea that Black people did not deserve to live in wealthy neighborhoods or that Black people would destroy the moral fabric of "White neighborhoods" if they were allowed to live there supported segregated housing policies, like exclusionary zoning, which still exist. People of color, like Black people, are still more likely to live in poorer, strategically disadvantaged neighborhoods when compared to White people,[24] and it stems from a legacy of discriminatory housing policies. Keeping Black people from safe and advantaged neighborhoods is exactly what it means to intentionally keep Black people from the social determinants of health, including those needed for restful sleep. Housing is an important social determinant of health, but given housing's racist distribution, housing is often a pathway for poor sleep for Black people. Housing can also determine our proximity to pollution, which is also a social determinant of health inequitably experienced by economically poor people and people of color, including Black people.

Environmental Racism

Climate change and environmental toxins and their effects on humans, animals, and our natural environment are a concern for many people. Policies and regulations that ban plastic bags in grocery stores, require our vehicles to undergo yearly emissions tests, or limits to the toxins that large factories can emit are all in an effort to slow the progression of climate change. Indeed there are many other actions that individuals and businesses voluntarily take and are forced to take to protect our environment. Despite some policy and behavioral changes though, we all continue to feel the effects of climate change and environmental changes from higher or lower than normal seasonal temperatures to an increase in natural disasters like tornadoes and hurricanes. Many people are rightly concerned for our planet and for its inhabitants and wish more was being done. What makes how we treat our environment an even more pressing issue is that economically poor people and people of color, specifically Indigenous, Latinx, Asian, and Black people, are the most affected by a polluted environment. This includes the harm environmental toxins pose to overall health and sleep health.

A 2021 study found that regardless of their income or which state they live in, all people of color in the United States have higher rates of exposure to air toxins. The toxins are hazardous particles, known as particulate matter 2.5 (PM 2.5), which represents the particles' diameter of less than 2.5 micrometers or less than 1/13 of a strand of human hair.[25] PM 2.5 are small enough to enter our lungs and cause respiratory and heart disease and are known to cause premature death. Black people, in particular, have greater than average exposure to PM 2.5 emitted from fourteen sources identified by the Environmental Protection Agency (EPA) including construction, gas vehicles, road dust, and commercial cooking as well as from other sources. White people have slightly higher than average rates of exposure to air toxins from sources like agriculture and coal plants, but overall, their exposure to air pollutants is less than people of color's rates of exposure. This disparity, often referred to as environmental injustice or environmental racism, reveals the ways that environmental hazards disproportionately jeopardize Black people's health. One reason Black people are more affected by environmental toxins is because of the sources of toxins. Toxic sources like toxic landfills are disproportionately located near where Black people live, work, and go to school and are very unlikely to be located in affluent and/or predominantly White neighborhoods.[26]

At first glance, exposure to environmental toxins may seem like just a threat to overall health and not like an obvious threat to sleep. Social determinants of health like access to clean air, however, are also social determinants of sleep. As such, environmental toxins are a pathway to poor sleep through at least two main routes—one being that exposure to environmental toxins introduces and/or exacerbates illness into our lives. For example, Black and Indigenous children have almost double the rate of asthma than White children.[27] Black children are also four times as likely to have asthma related hospitalizations and ten times as likely to have asthma related deaths than White children.[28] Children of color also have higher rates of exposure to environmental toxins like carbon monoxide and lead while at home and while at school.[29] We cannot talk about racial disparities in asthma without talking about air toxins as possible contributors. And illness often comes with a physical, mental, and financial price tag for ourselves and for those charged with our care like our spouses, parents, and family members. By introducing sickness and stress into our lives, environmental toxins also jeopardize sleep. We can imagine how children whose asthma is worsened by air pollutants may not sleep well and how their parents might have their sleep affected by worry for their sick children or worry about having the financial resources to pay for their children's health care.

Secondly, environmental toxins complicate our relationship with our homes by making our homes sources of pollution and illness, and thus sleeplessness. For Black people, their higher than normal exposure to environmental toxins turn their homes into dangerous and unhealthy places to live and sleep. And when we look at their specific experiences with soil, air, and water toxins, all throughout the United States, we can see how environmental toxins pose a threat to sleep health.

"Cancer Alley"

In Louisiana, between Baton Rouge and New Orleans, there are mostly all Black communities that have been nicknamed "Cancer Alley."[30] These communities were given this insidious nickname because of its numerous oil and gas plants and other industrial facilities that emit toxins, including plants from popular companies like Shell and ExxonMobil. This part of Louisiana is also known as "Cancer Alley" because its residents have higher than average rates of cancer. In the 1980s and 1990s when Black people were seeking social mobility and their piece of the American dream, they bought homes in this area not knowing that the homes were built on top of toxic landfills. But after they and their family and neighbors starting getting sick and the cancer diagnoses started rolling in, the residents knew that they were being poisoned by their homes. The residents knew they were living in "Cancer Alley" well before researchers and government agencies started declaring their air among the deadliest air in America.

Jesse Perkins lives in "Cancer Alley." Perkins is a Black man who, like many other Black people in the 1980s, bought a home thinking that he was creating a better life for himself. In 1988 Jesse Perkins bought his first home in Gordon Plaza, a housing development built with the help of federal funding and marketed to middle-class Black families in New Orleans. What Perkins did not know was that his home was built on a toxic dump. For fifty years the land beneath his home and other homes, businesses, elementary schools, and senior living homes was used to spray toxins on and incinerate medical, municipal, and industrial waste. In the 1980s and 1990s testing done on the soil revealed about 150 harmful contaminants, including cancer-causing toxins like arsenic.

A 2019 study found that in the area surrounding Gordon Plaza, 745 people per 1 million were diagnosed with cancer, which is higher than the Louisiana state average of 489 people per 1 million. Marilyn Amar, a sixty-nine-year-old Black woman who has lived in Gordon Plaza since 1990, is one of the residents of "Cancer Alley" who has been diagnosed with cancer. Amar attributes her breast cancer, as well as her son's mysterious childhood illnesses and intestinal surgery to vegetables in her backyard garden grown in toxic soil. Amar is just one of the people whose lives have been altered by environmental toxins and deceit. Other Louisiana residents, whose homes are surrounded by factories and foul smelling air, attribute their cancer to the toxins from the oil and gas facilities in the areas as well.[31]

In 1997, the EPA dug up 2 feet of topsoil in parts of Gordon Plaza that did not have any buildings or other structures built on top of it. The agency placed the equivalent of a net on top of toxic soil, placed noncontaminated soil on top of the net, and told residents this would make their neighborhoods safe. Even though the EPA did not place netting and noncontaminated soil on land underneath roads, schools, homes, or any land with structures on top of it, the efforts they did put in to fix the problem do not do much for Gordon Plaza's residents. A net and some new soil does not fix their toxic soil and cancer problem. The net and new soil only act as a slight barrier between toxic soil and the new non-toxic soil; it is a warning for anyone who chooses to dig into the soil in the future. It does not remove any toxins from the soil in the freestanding areas and it does not remove toxins from the soil underneath their homes, schools, and businesses. As Marilyn Amar put it: "The toxins are still there. They did a cover-up, not a clean-up." Feeling misled and lied to, Gordon Plaza's almost all Black residents want their local government to help relocate them so they can live in safer homes; as of 2020, though, the city of New Orleans has refused to help. In fact, more oil and gas plants, known sources of environmental toxins, are planned to be built in the mostly poor and Black neighborhoods whose air is already deemed to be some of the most dangerous in the country.[32] Louisiana residents are organizing, protesting, and taking other legal action to prevent more facilities from being built, but so far the local government is not budging, citing jobs and economic growth for Louisiana as a benefit of the plants.

The almost all Black residents of Reserve, Louisiana have had similar experiences living amongst industrial facilities. In 2015 the EPA found that because of the air pollutants in the area's air, many of its residents' risk of cancer is fifty times higher than the national average. In fact almost every home in Reserve has had someone die from cancer.[33] Similarly, the mostly Black (and Latinx) and economically poor Fifth Ward in Houston, Texas are also experiencing higher-than-normal rates of cancer from environmental toxins, like arsenic, emitted by the railroads located throughout their neighborhood.[34] People in these areas are disproportionately experiencing illness and death because of environmental toxins. Sheena Dedmond, a thirty-five-year-old Black resident of Gordon Plaza (her home was once owned by her mother), for example, saw her mother die from cancer, her father live with a brain tumor, and her neighbors diagnosed with cancer or other life-threatening diseases. Living in polluted areas like Gordon Plaza, Reserve, and the Fifth Ward, according to Dedmond, "It's not just that we're living on top of cancer-causing chemicals, it's like living in a cemetery. We're just waiting to die."

The story of Gordon Plaza, Reserve, and the Fifth Ward's plight with environmental toxins, is an example of the systemic ways healthy housing is frequently withheld from Black people, but they are just a few examples among many. It might be easy to suggest to the individuals who live in these neighborhoods that they move to homes in safer neighborhoods. One might say "well, if your neighborhood is poisoning you, move to another neighborhood." Despite side-stepping the moral problem of companies poisoning mostly Black people, people of color, and poor people, this response also ignores the economic predicament many of the people in these neighborhoods find themselves. If the people in these neighborhoods could move, we can be certain that they would. In fact, many families have moved out of these neighborhoods. For many of the other families, however, it is not an option to move. Moving is expensive, purchasing or renting a new home is also expensive. Also, many residents in these toxic areas own their home and it is unlikely that they would be able to find someone willing to buy their home given that they now know the home is built on or near toxic land. Simply put, most of the Black residents in these neighborhoods are trapped in these toxic areas and need assistance to leave. But instead of the responsible parties helping them out of the predicament they created, the residents are met with resistance and closed doors.

Taking a look at how environmental toxins predominantly affect poor people and people of color highlights the reality that a person's zip code can determine their health; if we live in zip codes in affluent areas we are more likely to have better health, but if we live in zip codes in poor areas we are more likely to have poor health.[35] In fact, some researchers estimate that up to 60 percent of our health is determined by where we live, rather than our genes, because where we live is connected to our access to social determinants of health.[36] Although, some researchers may not agree with this exact percentage, the point is that a large portion of our health is determined by factors external to our own bodies, meaning our health can be jeopardized by external factors. For example, social stability is a social determinant of health that confers health and wellbeing and environmental pollutants can destabilize the health of entire communities. The unfortunate truth is that wealthy people, and many White people, do not live in areas with the highest levels of pollution or where gas and oil plants are located, whereas many Black people and other people of color call these facilities "neighbors." And if zip codes can determine our health and our proximity to facilities that contribute to poor health, they certainly can determine sleep given the intertwined nature of overall health, our social health, and sleep.

It is not difficult to imagine the mechanisms by which environmental toxins might affect sleep. If people are worried that just by living in their homes or eating the vegetables they have grown in their own backyard gardens can quite literally kill themselves and their families, sleep might be elusive. Besides worrying about potential toxins, the actual toxins in their neighborhood also affect sleep quality. In fact, the data tells us that Black people, like Kimberly Turner (as told in the chapter opening), have the highest rates of breathing-related sleep disorders, such as sleep apnea, which disrupts their sleep.[37] Neither inferior respiratory systems nor bad luck explain Black people's higher rates of breathing-related sleep disorders. Rather the social consequences of being Black, including having lesser income, lesser access to healthy foods and recreation, poorer housing, and more exposure to environmental toxins contribute to Black people's sleep disorders and their lesser sleep quality.

Having to fight to live in healthy and safe neighborhoods is also a tax on the people living in these polluted areas. The effort that Black people in these neighborhoods and towns must put forth to fight for visibility, to be heard by businesses that brought the toxins into their homes and the government officials who ignore them, can also make quality sleep elusive. But they continue to take on the extra burden of literally fighting for their lives and fighting for their local governments to care about their health because their lives and the lives of their families and neighbors depend on it. The people who live in Cancer Alley, Reserve, the Fifth Ward and the many neighborhoods like it across America are the faces behind the data on environmental toxins' unequal effects on Black communities. They are the faces behind environmental toxins making homes, the places where people sleep, dangerous and not conducive to proper health and sleep. But unfortunately, environmental racism is just one pathway to sleeplessness among many others, including racism-related vigilance.

Remaining Vigilant

Racial discrimination has been shown to impact the quality of sleep Black people receive.[38] A study conducted by Tomfohr and colleagues used "The Scale of Ethnic Experience" to determine perceived discrimination, which is a measurement of an individual's belief that members of their race experience discrimination. From the study, researchers concluded that racial discrimination was a factor associated with how well Black people sleep.[39] For Black participants, their experiences with racial discrimination were linked with more time in light sleep stages than deep sleep stages. The researchers believe this is because of racism-related vigilance, which is a way to measure race-related stress.[40]

Racism-related vigilance is the stress that Black people experience when they anticipate and prepare for racist behaviors from institutions or individuals they encounter in their everyday life. For example, Black people may employ racism-related vigilance while shopping at affluent retail stores because they expect to be followed by staff members who think that because they are Black they will steal the store's merchandise. Since racism is intertwined with the experience of being Black in America, simply because of racism's prevalence in our country, racism-related vigilance is arguably a necessary part of surviving being Black.

Race-related vigilance is another example of a burden that jeopardizes Black people's mental and psychological health that White people do not have simply because they are White. Race related vigilance is a way of life for many Black people in ways that it is not for White people. For instance, in an interview one Black woman stated how racism-related vigilance operates in her life:[41]

> I feel as though most of the time I find myself being in a guarded position or somewhat on the defense. I somewhat stay prepared to be discriminated against because I never know when it's going to happen to me.

While living their normal lives, Black people must always stay alert for racist behavior and attitudes because they too easily can turn into race-motivated violence. Not practicing race-related vigilance can often mean the difference between life or death. An example of this can be seen in Christian Cooper's 2020 experiences while visiting Central Park.[42]

Christian Cooper, a Black man, was bird watching in Central Park in New York City when he asked Amy Cooper (no relation to Christian Cooper), a White woman, to follow park rules and put a leash on her unleashed dog. In response Amy stated that she would call the cops and tell them that an African American man was threatening her life. Christian began to film her as she called the cops and made the false claim that he was threatening to harm her. When his cell phone video of his encounter with Amy went viral, many Black people were relieved that this incident did not end with Christian being falsely imprisoned or killed by responding police officers because that outcome has happened many times before. In fact, that is likely why Amy called the police and created this false narrative; she wanted Christian to be legally punished for what she believed was his transgression—a Black man asking her to abide by the same rules as everyone else. As Christian said after the event: "Unfortunately we live in an era with things like Ahmaud Arbery [a Black man shot and killed by two White men while he was out jogging days after Cooper's incident], where Black men are seen as targets. This woman thought she could exploit that to her advantage, and I wasn't having it."

As Christian states, Amy wanted to weaponize her social status as a White woman and use it against Christian's status as a Black man, creating another instance of the contentious and often deadly relationship between Black people, particularly Black men, and the police. Amy was relying on the racist and false narrative of Black male aggression to her advantage, to paint herself as a victim and the Black man as a perpetrator of harm against her. The narrative that Black men are excessively aggressive and dangerous, particularly to White women, making Black men a threat to them, is a narrative that has been used and continues to be used to falsely accuse Black men of crimes against White people.[43] As such, race-related vigilance can be imperative to Black people's survival and freedom from false imprisonment. If Christian had not participated in race-related vigilance and recorded his interactions with Amy as proof of his innocence and her wrongdoing, the ending of this story may not have ended with Christian's survival. Without his quick thinking, this story could have ended like so many others, with his death and his name becoming a hashtag on social media. Making Christian's story more incredible is that hours later, George Floyd's encounter with Minneapolis police officers ended with his murder, which sparked worldwide protests against institutional racism against Black people and police brutality.[44] Floyd's story, unfortunately, did not end like Christian's.

Race-related vigilance, like staying alert for racism and having to record their encounters with racist people to prove their innocence, puts an additional burden on Black people that White people do not have to worry about. The privilege of not worrying about whether their skin color will encourage racially motivated behavior, including murder, is not afforded to Black people. One Black woman made a similar observation about her own behavior:

> [One problem with] being Black in America is that you have to spend so much time thinking about stuff that most White people just don't even have to think about. I worry when I get pulled over by a cop . . . I worry when I walk into a store that someone is going to think that I am shoplifting. And I have to worry about that because I am not free to ignore it.[45]

This woman expresses the lack of freedom that comes with being Black because of the mental alertness that she, and most other Black people, must constantly possess. And since racism is not bound by class, income, education (Christian Cooper is a Harvard University graduate), or neighborhood, it is a part of the Black experience regardless of other social characteristics a person may possess.

Race related vigilance is akin to what scholars call the "autonomy problem." The "autonomy problem" occurs when people feel they do not have complete control over the daily happenings in their lives, nor the overall outcome of their lives because of external factors, such as the effects of racism.[46] Race-related vigilance stems from a lack of control over whether people will judge, treat harshly, verbally and physically harm, and/or criminalize Black individuals any time they want and feeling like there is nothing that Black people can do about it. Even the experience of witnessing racial discrimination, either in person or for instance in social media videos of race motivated police killings of unarmed Black people, can produce feelings of having no autonomy over our lives. Race-related vigilance and the autonomy problem are manifestations of feeling unsafe in America because of its culture of anti-Black racial discrimination.

The stress of knowing that at any moment a Black individual could be subject to the effects of racism, including murder by citizens or police officers, takes control away from Black individuals. It takes away their sense of security, all of which is needed for restful sleep. Being Black in America comes with stresses that other people just do not have, and it contributes to racial disparities in sleep between White and Black people. Anticipating and experiencing emotionally distressing events interrupts our sleep.[47] This is supported by much research, which shows that distressing race-related thoughts and feelings interrupt sleep, contributing to Black people getting less quality sleep.[48]

Moleendo Stewart, a Black man who lives in Brooklyn, believes that discrimination is partly to blame for his sleep troubles: "As a Black person in America, even if you succeed in terms of education, you still have to deal with the inherent inequality of society.[49] I don't blame it on the majority-that's just simplistic. But in general, it's not a fair thing, and you stress because of that." Stewart's thoughts on his sleep behavior echo the autonomy problem and its effects on Black people's sleep health. Stewart's thoughts about his sleep health also reinforce the data that shows when discrimination is removed from the equation, researchers have found that the sleep health of Black and White people looks roughly the same.[50] Racism and racial discrimination creates another hurdle for Black people looking for a restful night's sleep. The mental and physical toll racism puts on Black people's sleep should not be underestimated.

Sleep Hygiene

Sleep hygiene is advice, or tips for developing good sleep habits, often given to people by health care providers and public health agencies.[51] Having good sleep hygiene is supposed to equate to getting quality sleep and being well rested throughout the day. There are many tips for getting better sleep, but here are some of the most prominent tips:[52]

1. Go to bed and wake up at the same time each night and morning.
2. Exercise regularly during the day.
3. Remove electronic devices like TVs and cellular phones from the room.
4. Eat proper meals.
5. Make sure your bedroom is the right temperature, dark, and free from noise.

Sleep hygiene encourages us to make behavioral and lifestyle changes if we cannot sleep. It also tries to deter us from poor sleep hygiene like using our phones in bed, napping during the day, or staying up very late at night.[53]

Sleep hygiene requires us to have access to the social determinants of health like food security, stable housing, stable employment and income, and access to safe places for recreation in addition to social determinants of sleep like the freedom to choose where and how we sleep. For example, to "exercise regularly during the day" we must have the money to pay for a gym membership or live in neighborhoods safe enough for exercising outdoors. Sleep hygiene's starting point is the assumption that people have access to the social determinants of health needed for proper sleep. But some Black people often lack many of the social determinants of health that sleep hygiene requires. Telling people who are not sleeping that they just need better sleep hygiene assumes people have the social determinants of health and just need to better regulate them for better sleep health. Sleep hygiene targets individual behaviors, but addressing sleeplessness requires us to address systemic social inequities that prevent people from having the resources they need for proper sleep.

Sleep hygiene is ultimately privileged advice. It is idealism and it does not help people who do not live under ideal conditions. As Charles Mills asks, "*cui bono*" or "'for whose benefit' does it serve to pretend like our life is ideal and ignore oppression and discrimination?"[54]

> Can it possibly serve the interests of women to ignore female subordination, represent the family as ideal, and pretend that women have been treated as equal persons? Obviously not. Can it possibly serve the interests of people of color to ignore the centuries of White supremacy, and to pretend that a discourse originally structured around White normativity now substantively, as against just terminologically, includes them? Obviously not. Can it possibly serve the interests of the poor and the working class to ignore the ways in which an increasingly inequitable class society imposes economic constraints that limit their normal freedoms, and undermine their formal equality before the law? Obviously not.

Similarly, when they are not sleeping well, it does not serve Black people's interests to pretend that they live under ideal circumstances. Sleep hygiene does not account for people's lack of access to what they need for sleep health. Black people's sleeplessness is influenced by their inadequate housing, racial discrimination, and exposure to environmental toxins, among other deficient resources. Sleep hygiene does not account for structural inequities and racism's disproportionate influence on Black people's lives, which could be affecting their sleep. If a person lives in a food desert or does not have enough money to afford food, telling them that that if they would just eat regularly, they will sleep better does nothing to address the source of their sleeplessness. Some researchers have found that even when Black people do not have sleep disorders, they are still at a higher risk for sleeplessness because they do not have proper access to the social determinants of health.[55] This is because the social determinants of health are the social determinants of sleep. Inequities in social determinants of health mean less sleep. The consequences of inequities in social determinants of health are racial disparities in sleep, with Black people, once again, on the losing end.

Sleep hygiene is an example of how medicine and public health organizations fail to consider the lived experience of being Black and its effects on Black people's health. Clinicians and medical organizations pedaling sleep hygiene is also an example of how socially disadvantaged people can be blamed for their own poor health.[56] Instead of using what we know about racial disparities in sleep to create racially aware sleep advice, sleep hygiene is often unhelpful, generic advice that can only help the privileged few.

Bedtimes and Cultural Determinants

One of the most prominent sleep hygiene tips is to regulate our bedtimes, that is, make sure that we are going to bed at the same time as often as possible. But sleep hygiene does not take into account that what time people go to sleep can be a matter of cultural difference. For the most part, the cultural differences between Black and White people that could help explain some racial disparities in sleep amount to scholars' speculations, but they are worth mentioning. One speculation is that differences in childhood bedtimes may influence racial disparities in sleep. The idea is that Black children are less likely to have set bedtimes than White children. So perhaps this behavior set the trend for Black adults to not have set bedtimes as well, resulting in them going to sleep later in the evening when compared to White adults. And when people do not have set bedtimes they can experience sleeplessness.

Another speculation that comes up in the literature is that perhaps Black adults are reporting their sleep troubles to health care providers less often than White adults and instead seeking remedies elsewhere, such as discussing their sleep issues with friends, family, or spiritual advisors. Although Black people as a group do tend to be family-oriented and religious, when considering this possible explanation for racial disparities in sleep, we have to consider whether this explanation places the blame on Black people for their sleeplessness. In other words, is this speculation saying that it is Black people's fault that they are not sleeping because they are not going to see a health care provider for care? As this chapter suggests, we have to consider that if Black people are not going to see a health care provider, why aren't they? Is there some barrier—social, economic, or cultural—that stops them from seeing a health care provider? And if they are going to see a health care provider, what kind of care are they receiving once they do? When considering why Black people do not sleep very well, we have to examine barriers and social inequities that stand in their way.

If there are cultural differences such as differing bedtimes and where Black people choose to seek help for sleeplessness, or other differences that have yet to be determined that can help explain racial disparities in sleep, these suggested differences show us that we have to examine the social context of racial disparities in sleep. Situating sleeplessness among Black people within a social context makes sleeplessness not a moral failure. Context provides a deeper understanding of racial disparities in sleep and an understanding that the reasons may not always be that Black people have failed to take the appropriate steps to get proper sleep.

Conclusion

Black people do not sleep poorly because Black people are more biologically prone to sleep disorders or are on their phones during the night more than White people. Black people's experiences with sleeplessness exist because of differing access to social determinants of health, which are also social determinants of sleep. Black people are disproportionately affected by environmental pollution, have lesser access to proper housing than White people, and practice-race related vigilance in their everyday lives. Black people have differing access to social determinants of health largely because of the ways their race, gender, and class make them vulnerable to abuse and oppression from the institutions meant to protect citizens and their health. But because of their Blackness they are not afforded these protections.

To eliminate the sleep gap between White and Black individuals we have to employ policies, regulations, and laws that dismantle institutions' racist and oppressive practices. For example, the laws that contribute to legal housing segregation must be reformed. We have to change the way we treat sleeplessness in Black people, namely by using the lived experiences of Blackness to treat Black patients. Because of the importance of sleep to our overall health, racial disparities in sleep should be viewed as a troubling and unjust aspect of our culture. And for anyone interested in public health, how much and how often Black people sleep should be at the forefront of discussions of justice.

Discussion Questions

1. When you cannot sleep how does it affect your life? How does this impact how you think about Black people's sleeplessness?
2. Why should we care about how much Black people sleep?
3. What can clinicians do differently to help their Black patients suffering from sleeplessness?
4. Can you think of any other social or political determinants contributing to Black people's sleeplessness?
5. What are some other examples of policies and laws that institutions could create and enforce that would mitigate or even end racial disparities in sleep?

Acknowledgments

A person like me, one of the handful of Black women philosophers and bioethicists, does not get to the point of being able to write a book like this without help. To the family, friends, teachers, and colleagues who early on in my life and throughout my career believed I could do great things, encouraged me, and mentored me, thank you.

A special thank you to my mom and biggest cheerleader, Kimberly. And to my grandmother Anita, who was the first person to tell me that I would be a writer: I wish you could be here to see this, but I felt your presence as I wrote this book. To my family and my best friends, whom I love dearly, thank you for your unwavering support and love. To Tanisha, my sister/cousin, thanks for always cheering me on.

To my colleagues at the McGovern Center for Humanities and Ethics at UTHealth Houston, thank you for your kindness, for reading drafts, and for your overall support. A special thanks to Rev. Dr. Nathan Carlin who was the first person to tell me I could write a book like this and get it published, long before I believed I could. Thank you for always being in my corner.

To the colleagues and reviewers who read drafts and pushed me to make the book better, thank you. To the many scholars who invited me to share my work with your institutions and with your students and to the lecture attendees who asked me questions that made my work better, I appreciate you. You gave me a safe space to work out my thoughts and piece together this book and I am very grateful. To my students who engaged in thoughtful discussion with me about these topics, I learned so much from your willingness to grow as scholars and caregivers and be better physicians to your Black patients.

I have much appreciation for the Charles Alston estate for allowing me to use Mr. Alston's important and moving piece of African American art on the cover of this book.

Thank you to Faith Fletcher and Patrick Smith who spent two long days in Houston workshopping this book. Your feedback was invaluable. Thank you, Esther and Shannon for your assistance with the bibliography and index. And thank you to series editors Sean Valles and Quill Kukla for your feedback and support. Thank you to Lucy Randall for believing in this project.

Lastly, what makes this book special to me are the stories from Black people. The stories give the book character and depth and it would have been impossible to write this book without them. To the people who shared their most intimate stories of pain, fear, abuse, and illness, thank you for your vulnerability. Thank you for sharing this part of you so that I and others may learn. I hope that I have done your stories justice and treated you with compassion.

Notes

Introduction

1. Steve Almasy, "Detroit Bus Driver Jason Hargrove Dies Days after Making Video about Coughing Passenger," CNN, May 3, 2020, https://www.cnn.com/2020/04/03/us/detroit-bus-driver-dies-coronavirus-trnd/index.html.
2. CDC, "Covid Data Tracker," Centers for Disease Control and Prevention, May 31, 2022, https://covid.cdc.gov/covid-data-tracker/#demographics
3. Domenico Cucinotta and Maurizio Vanelli, "WHO Declares COVID-19 a Pandemic," *Acta Bio-Medica: Atenei Parmensis* 91, no. 1 (March 19, 2020): 157–60, https://doi.org/10.23750/abm.v91i1.9397.
4. CDC, "Hospitalization and Death by Race/Ethnicity," Centers for Disease Control and Prevention, February 11, 2020, https://www.cdc.gov/coronavirus/2019-ncov/covid-data/investigations-discovery/hospitalization-death-by-race-ethnicity.html.
5. CDC, "Health Equity Considerations & Racial & Ethnic Minority Groups," Centers for Disease Control and Prevention, January 25, 2022, https://www.cdc.gov/coronavirus/2019-ncov/community/health-equity/race-ethnicity.html.
6. American Medical Association, "Advancing Health Equity: A Guide to Language, Narrative and Concepts," 2021, https://www.ama-assn.org/system/files/ama-aamc-equity-guide.pdf.
7. Richard Rothstein, *The Color of Law: A Forgotten History of How Our Government Segregated America*, first edition (New York; London: Liveright Publishing Corporation, a division of W. W. Norton & Company, 2017).
8. John Hoberman, *Black and Blue: The Origins and Consequences of Medical Racism* (Los Angeles: University of California Press, 2012).
9. Heckler, Margaret M, Report of the Secretary's Task Force Report on Black and Minority Health, vol. 1: Executive Summary, U.S. Department of Health and Human Services, 1985.
10. Kimberle Crenshaw, "Demarginalizing the Intersection of Race and Sex: A Black Feminist Critique of Antidiscrimination Doctrine, Feminist Theory and Antiracist Politics," no. 1 (1989): 31.

11. R. Cooper and R. David, "The Biological Concept of Race and Its Application to Public Health and Epidemiology," *Journal of Health Politics, Policy and Law* 11, no. 1 (1986): 97–116, https://doi.org/10.1215/03616878-11-1-97; R. Witzig, "The Medicalization of Race: Scientific Legitimization of a Flawed Social Construct," *Annals of Internal Medicine* 125, no. 8 (October 15, 1996): 675–79, https://doi.org/10.7326/0003-4819-125-8-199610150-00008; Audrey Smedley and Brian D. Smedley, "Race as Biology Is Fiction, Racism as a Social Problem Is Real: Anthropological and Historical Perspectives on the Social Construction of Race," *The American Psychologist* 60, no. 1 (January 2005): 16–26, https://doi.org/10.1037/0003-066X.60.1.16.

12. Ijeoma Oluo, *So You Want to Talk about Race*, first edition (New York: Seal Press, 2018).

13. Edward Baptiste, *The Half Has Never Been Told: Slavery and the Making of American Capitalism* (New York: Basic Books, 2014)

14. Terence Keel, *Divine Variations: How Christian Thought Became Racial Science* (Stanford: Stanford University Press, 2018)

15. Harriet Washington, *Medical Apartheid: The Dark History of Medical Experimentation on Black Americans from Colonial Times to the Present* (New York: First Anchor Books, 2006), 46.

16. Carl C. Bell and Harshad Mehta, "The Misdiagnosis of Black Patients with Manic Depressive Illness," *Journal of the National Medical Association* 72, no. 2 (February 1980): 141–45.

17. N. Krieger, "Shades of Difference: Theoretical Underpinnings of the Medical Controversy on Black/White Differences in the United States, 1830–1870," *International Journal of Health Services: Planning, Administration, Evaluation* 17, no. 2 (1987): 259–78, https://doi.org/10.2190/DBY6-VDQ8-HME8-ME3R.

18. "Encyclopedia of Social Problems," in One Drop Rule, February 5, 2022, https://us.sagepub.com/en-us/nam/encyclopedia-of-social-problems/book229800.

19. Nikki Khanna, "'If You're Half Black, You're Just Black': Reflected Appraisals and the Persistence of the One-Drop Rule," *The Sociological Quarterly* 51, no. 1 (December 1, 2016): 96–121, https://doi.org/10.1111/j.1533-8525.2009.01162.x.

20. F. James Davis, *Who Is Black? One Nation's Definition* (University Park: Pennsylvania State University Press, 1991).

21. Dorothy Roberts, *Fatal Invention: How Science, Politics, and Big Business Re-create Race in the Twenty-First Century* (New York: New Press,

2011); Tukufu Zuberi, *Thicker than Blood: How Racial Statistics Lie* (Minneapolis: University of Minnesota Press, 2001).

22. National Human Genome Research Institute, "Genetics vs. Genomics Fact Sheet," September 7, 2018, https://www.genome.gov/about-genom ics/fact-sheets/Genetics-vs-Genomics.

23. MedlinePlus Genetics, "Sickle Cell Disease," National Library of Medicine, August 18, 2020, https://medlineplus.gov/genetics/condition/sickle-cell-disease/; U.S National Heart, Lung, and Blood Institute, "Sickle Cell Disease," September 1, 2020, https://www.nhlbi.nih.gov/health-topics/sic kle-cell-disease.

24. David R. Williams, "African-American Health: The Role of the Social Environment," *Journal of Urban Health: Bulletin of the New York Academy of Medicine* 75, no. 2 (June 1998): 300–21, https://doi.org/10.1007/BF0 2345099.

25. Michael Yudell et al., "SCIENCE AND SOCIETY. Taking Race out of Human Genetics," *Science* 351, no. 6273 (February 5, 2016): 564–65, https://doi.org/10.1126/science.aac4951.

26. Keisha Ray, "Intersectionality and the Dangers of White Empathy When Treating Black Patients," *Bioethics Today*, 2017, https://bioethicstoday.org/ blog/intersectionality-and-the-dangers-of-white-empathy-when-treat ing-black-patients/.

27. Oluo, *So You Want to Talk about Race*, 26–27.

28. American Medical Association, 2021.

29. Lorraine T Dean et al., "What Structural Racism Is (or Is Not) and How to Measure It: Clarity for Public Health and Medical Researchers," *American Journal of Epidemiology*, 2022

30. WHO (World Health Organization). 2012. *What Are the Social Determinants of Health?* Available at: http://www.who.int/social_deter minants/sdh_definition/en/

31. Jacob B. Pierce et al., "Association of Childhood Psychosocial Environment With a 30-Year Cardiovascular Disease Incidence and Mortality in Middle Age," *Journal of the American Heart Association* 9, no. 9 (28 April 2020)

32. R. J. Blendon et al., "Access to Medical Care for Black and White Americans. A Matter of Continuing Concern," *JAMA* 261, no. 2 (January 13, 1989): 278–81.

33. Lauren Hale et al., "Perceived Neighborhood Quality, Sleep Quality, and Health Status: Evidence from the Survey of the Health of Wisconsin," *Social Science & Medicine* (1982) 79 (February 2013): 16–22, https://doi. org/10.1016/j.socscimed.2012.07.021; Douglas Quenqua, "How Well You

Sleep May Hinge on Race," *The New York Times*, August 20, 2012, sec. Health, https://www.nytimes.com/2012/08/21/health/how-well-you-sleep-may-hinge-on-race.html.

34. Craig Evan Pollack et al., "Should Health Studies Measure Wealth? A Systematic Review," *American Journal of Preventive Medicine* 33, no. 3 (September 2007): 250–64, https://doi.org/10.1016/j.amepre.2007.04.033; D. R. Williams, "Race, Socioeconomic Status, and Health. The Added Effects of Racism and Discrimination," *Annals of the New York Academy of Sciences* 896 (1999): 173–88, https://doi.org/10.1111/j.1749-6632.1999. tb08114.x.

35. David R. Williams and Toni D. Rucker, "Understanding and Addressing Racial Disparities in Health Care," *Health Care Financing Review* 21, no. 4 (2000): 75–90.

36. Margaret T. Hicken et al., "'Every Shut Eye, Ain't Sleep': The Role of Racism-Related Vigilance in Racial/Ethnic Disparities in Sleep Difficulty," *Race and Social Problems* 5, no. 2 (June 1, 2013): 100–112, https://doi.org/10.1007/s12552-013-9095-9.

37. Oluwaseun A. Akinseye et al., "Sleep as a Mediator in the Pathway Linking Environmental Factors to Hypertension: A Review of the Literature," *International Journal of Hypertension* 2015 (2015): 926414, https://doi.org/10.1155/2015/926414; Aaron D. Laposky, Eve Van Cauter, and Ana V. Diez-Roux, "Reducing Health Disparities: The Role of Sleep Deficiency and Sleep Disorders," *Sleep Medicine* 18 (February 2016): 3–6, https://doi.org/10.1016/j.sleep.2015.01.007.

38. Kelly M. Hoffman et al., "Racial Bias in Pain Assessment and Treatment Recommendations, and False Beliefs about Biological Differences between Blacks and Whites," *Proceedings of the National Academy of Sciences of the United States of America* 113, no. 16 (April 19, 2016): 4296–4301, https://doi.org/10.1073/pnas.1516047113.

39. Elizabeth A. Howell et al., "Black-White Differences in Severe Maternal Morbidity and Site of Care," *American Journal of Obstetrics and Gynecology* 214, no. 1 (January 2016): 122.e1–122.e7, https://doi.org/10.1016/j.ajog.2015.08.019.

40. Center for Disease Control and Prevention, "Breast Cancer Rates Among Black Women and White Women," December 19, 2018, https://www.cdc.gov/cancer/breast/statistics/trends_invasive.htm.

41. Leslie R. M. Hausmann et al., "Racial Disparities in the Monitoring of Patients on Chronic Opioid Therapy," *Pain* 154, no. 1 (January 2013): 46–52, https://doi.org/10.1016/j.pain.2012.07.034; Jana M. Mossey, "Defining

Racial and Ethnic Disparities in Pain Management," *Clinical Orthopaedics and Related Research* 469, no. 7 (July 2011): 1859–70, https://doi.org/10.1007/s11999-011-1770-9.

42. Michael Sun et al., "Negative Patient Descriptors: Documenting Racial Bias in the Electronic Health Record: Study Examines Racial Bias in the Patient Descriptors Used in the Electronic Health Record.," *Health Affairs* 41, no. 2 (February 1, 2022): 203–11, https://doi.org/10.1377/hlth aff.2021.01423.

43. Corinne A. Riddell et al., "Trends in the Contribution of Major Causes of Death to the Black-White Life Expectancy Gap by US State," *Health & Place* 52 (July 2018): 85–100, https://doi.org/10.1016/j.healthplace.2018.04.003.

44. Howell et al., "Black-White Differences in Severe Maternal Morbidity and Site of Care."

45. Hoffman et al., "Racial Bias in Pain Assessment and Treatment Recommendations, and False Beliefs about Biological Differences between Blacks and Whites."

46. Natasha J. Williams et al., "Racial/Ethnic Disparities in Sleep Health and Health Care: Importance of the Sociocultural Context," *Sleep Health* 1, no. 1 (March 2015): 28–35, https://doi.org/10.1016/j.sleh.2014.12.004.

47. Chandra L. Jackson et al., "Racial Disparities in Short Sleep Duration by Occupation and Industry," *American Journal of Epidemiology* 178, no. 9 (November 1, 2013): 1442–51, https://doi.org/10.1093/aje/kwt159.

48. John Eligon and Robert Gebeloff, "Affluent and Black, and Still Trapped by Segregation," *The New York Times*, August 20, 2016, sec. U.S., https://www.nytimes.com/2016/08/21/us/milwaukee-segregation-wealthy-black-families.html.

49. Hale et al., "Perceived Neighborhood Quality, Sleep Quality, and Health Status."

Chapter 1

1. Nina Martin and Renee Montagne, "Nothing Protects Black Women From Dying in Pregnancy and Childbirth," *ProPublica*, 2017, https://www.propublica.org/article/nothing-protects-black-women-from-dying-in-pregnancy-and-childbirth?token=Q9-9suvCib74rpcNfQRtz25BI r6KF0ah.

2. "Maternal Mortality Rates in the United States, 2020," CDC, February 23, 2022, https://www.cdc.gov/nchs/data/hestat/maternal-mortality/2020/maternal-mortality-rates-2020.htm.

3. "Fact Sheet: The State of African American Women in the United States," Center for American Progress (blog), https://www.americanprogress.org/article/fact-sheet-the-state-of-african-american-women-in-the-united-states/.

4. Lisa Romero et al., "Reduced Disparities in Birth Rates Among Teens Aged 15–19 Years—United States, 2006–2007 and 2013–2014." *Morbidity and mortality weekly report 65*, no. 16 (April 29, 2016): 409–14.

5. Deirdre Cooper Owens and Sharla M. Fett. Black birthing and Infant Health: Historical Legacies of Slavery https://ajph.aphapublications.org/doi/pdf/10.2105/AJPH.2019.305243.

6. Dorothy Roberts, *Killing the Black Body*, 2nd ed. (New York: Vintage Books, 2017).

7. Roberts, 12.

8. Roberts, 59.

9. Julie Rose, "North Carolina Eugenics Victims Not Giving Up," NPR, August 17, 2012, sec. Law, https://www.npr.org/2012/08/17/158984357/north-carolina-eugenics-victims-plan-next-steps.

10. Roberts, *Killing the Black Body*, 90.

11. Harriet Washington, *Medical Apartheid: The Dark History of Medical Experimentation on Black Americans from Colonial Times to the Present* (New York: First Anchor Books, 2006).

12. Roberts, *Killing the Black Body*, 93.

13. Julia Naftulin, "Inside the Hidden Campaign to Forcibly Sterilize Thousands of Inmates in California Women's Prisons," *Insider*, https://www.insider.com/inside-forced-sterilizations-california-womens-prisons-documentary-2020-11.

14. Bill Chappell, "California's Prison Sterilizations Reportedly Echo Eugenics Era," NPR, July 9, 2013, sec. America, https://www.npr.org/sections/the-two-way/2013/07/09/200444613/californias-prison-sterilizations-reportedly-echoes-eugenics-era.

15. BBC, "New York: James Marion Sims Statue Removed From Central Park," BBC News, April 17, 2018, https://www.bbc.com/news/world-us-canada-43804725

16. Sarah Kuta, "Subjected to Painful Experiments and Forgotten, Enslaved 'Mothers of Gynecology' Are Honored With New Monument," *Smithsonian*, May 11, 2022, https://www.smithsonianmag.com/smart-news/mothers-of-gynecology-monument-honors-enslaved-women-180980064/

17. Brynn Holland, "The 'Father of Modern Gynecology' Performed Shocking Experiments on Enslaved Women," *HISTORY*, 2018, https://www.history.com/news/the-father-of-modern-gynecology-performed-shocking-experiments-on-slaves.

18. Washington, *Medical Apartheid*, 64; Roberts, *Killing the Black Body*.

19. Washington, *Medical Apartheid*, 64.

20. Karla F. C. Holloway, *Private Bodies, Public Texts: Race, Gender, and a Cultural Bioethics* (Durham, NC: Duke University Press, 2011).

21. Washington, *Medical Apartheid*, 65.

22. Washington, 59.

23. Washington, 69.

24. Colin A. Zestcott, Irene V. Blair, and Jeff Stone, "Examining the Presence, Consequences, and Reduction of Implicit Bias in Health Care: A Narrative Review," *Group Processes & Intergroup Relations: GPIR* 19, no. 4 (July 2016): 528–42, https://doi.org/10.1177/1368430216642029; Janice Sabin et al., "Physicians' Implicit and Explicit Attitudes about Race by MD Race, Ethnicity, and Gender," *Journal of Health Care for the Poor and Underserved* 20, no. 3 (August 2009): 896–913, https://doi.org/10.1353/hpu.0.0185; Meghan G. Bean et al., "Evidence of Nonconscious Stereotyping of Hispanic Patients by Nursing and Medical Students," *Nursing Research* 62, no. 5 (2013): 362–67, https://doi.org/10.1097/NNR.0b013e31829e02ec.

25. John Hoberman, *Black and Blue: The Origins and Consequences of Medical Racism* (Los Angeles: University of California Press, 2012), 141.

26. Roberts, *Killing the Black Body*; Hoberman, *Black and Blue: The Origins and Consequences of Medical Racism*.

27. Tina K. Sacks, *Invisible Visits: Black Middle Class Women in the American Healthcare System* (New York: Oxford University Press, 2019), 24.

28. Karen Ho, "The US Economic Recovery Is Skipping Black and Hispanic Women," *Quartz*, January 11, 2021, https://qz.com/1955437/black-and-hispanic-women-continued-to-lose-jobs-in-december/; Jaboa Lake, "The Pandemic Has Exacerbated Housing Instability for Renters of Color," Center for American Progress (blog), October 30, 2020, https://www.americanprogress.org/article/pandemic-exacerbated-housing-instability-renters-color/.

29. Melissa Victoria Harris-Perry, *Sister Citizen: Shame, Stereotypes, and Black Women in America; [for Colored Girls Who've Considered Politics When Being Strong Isn't Enough]* (New Haven, CT: Yale University Press, 2011); Roberts, *Killing the Black Body*.

30. Keisha Ray, "Blog—Black Women Are Dying in Disproportionate Numbers During and After Giving Birth and Not Even Celebrity Serena Williams Is Safe," *Bioethics Today*, January 16, 2018, https://bioethicsto day.org/blog/black-women-are-dying-in-disproportionate-numbers-dur ing-and-after-giving-birth-and-not-even-celebrity-serena-williams-is-safe/.

31. Pie Mumba, "Serena Williams' Birthing Scare Highlights Poor Black Maternal Health," Longevity, https://longevitylive.com/wellness/serena-williams-birthing-scare-highlights-poor-black-maternal-health/.

32. Jenn Barthole, "Black Maternal Health Week: Serena Williams Shares Her Near-Fatal Birthing Story," *Ebony*, April 11, 2022, https://www.ebony. com/lifestyle/serena-williams-shares-her-near-fatal-birthing-story1/

33. Kay Quinn, "Moms of Color Say They're Terrified of Dying in Childbirth and No One Is Listening," ksdk.com, October 24, 2018, https://www.ksdk. com/article/news/investigations/mothers-matter/moms-of-color-say-the yre-terrified-of-dying-in-childbirth-and-no-one-is-listening/63-607056 009; Nina Martin and Julia Belluz, "Lost Mothers," *ProPublica*, May 25, 2019, https://www.propublica.org/series/lost-mothers?token=aGn0c AzF1vcRrdeL0ElVR2hgvgtEPpJo.

34. "Racial and Ethnic Disparities Continue in Pregnancy-Related Deaths."

35. HBCU Editors, "Black Women Are Ranked the Most Educated Group by Race & Gender," HBCU Buzz (blog), March 4, 2014, https://hbcubuzz. com/2014/03/black-women-are-ranked-the-most-educated-group-by-race-gender/; Maria Guerra, "Fact Sheet: The State of African American Women in the United States," Center for American Progress (blog), November 7, 2013, https://www.americanprogress.org/article/fact-sheet-the-state-of-african-american-women-in-the-united-states/.

36. Shameka Poetry Thomas, "Trust Also Means Centering Black Women's Reproductive Health Narratives," *Hastings Center Report* 52, no. 2 (2022): S18–S21.

37. P. R. Lockhart, "What Serena Williams's Scary Childbirth Story Says about Medical Treatment of Black Women," *Vox*, January 11, 2018, https:// www.vox.com/identities/2018/1/11/16879984/serena-williams-childbi rth-scare-black-women.

38. Sacks, *Invisible Visits*, x.

39. Sacks, x.

40. Amy Roeder, "America Is Failing Its Black Mothers," *Harvard Public Health Magazine*, 2019, https://www.hsph.harvard.edu/magazine/magaz ine_article/america-is-failing-its-black-mothers/.

41. Arline T. Geronimus, "Black/White Differences in the Relationship of Maternal Age to Birthweight: A Population-Based Test of the Weathering Hypothesis," *Social Science & Medicine (1982)* 42, no. 4 (February 1996): 589–97, https://doi.org/10.1016/0277-9536(95)00159-x.

42. The American Institute of Stress, "Stress Effects," The American Institute of Stress (blog), n.d., https://www.stress.org/stress-effects.

43. Rodney Clark et al., "Racism as a Stressor for African Americans: A Biopsychosocial Model," *American Psychologist* 54, no. 10 (1999): 805–16, https://doi.org/10.1037/0003-066X.54.10.805; Jules P. Harrell, Sadiki Hall, and James Taliaferro, "Physiological Responses to Racism and Discrimination: An Assessment of the Evidence," *American Journal of Public Health* 93, no. 2 (February 2003): 243–48, https://doi.org/10.2105/AJPH.93.2.243.

44. N. Krieger, "The Ostrich, the Albatross, and Public Health: An Ecosocial Perspective—or Why an Explicit Focus on Health Consequences of Discrimination and Deprivation Is Vital for Good Science and Public Health Practice," *Public Health Reports* 116, no. 5 (2001): 419–23.

45. Michelle J. Sternthal, Natalie Slopen, and David R. Williams, "RACIAL DISPARITIES IN HEALTH: How Much Does Stress Really Matter?," *Du Bois Review: Social Science Research on Race* 8, no. 1 (May 15, 2011): 95–113, https://doi.org/10.1017/S1742058X11000087.

46. Arline T. Geronimus et al., "Do US Black Women Experience Stress-Related Accelerated Biological Aging?," *Human Nature (Hawthorne, N.Y.)* 21, no. 1 (March 10, 2010): 19–38, https://doi.org/10.1007/s12110-010-9078-0.

47. Masood A. Shammas, "Telomeres, Lifestyle, Cancer, and Aging," *Current Opinion in Clinical Nutrition and Metabolic Care* 14, no. 1 (January 2011): 28–34, https://doi.org/10.1097/MCO.0b013e32834121b1.

48. Roeder, "America Is Failing Its Black Mothers."

49. Shannon Sullivan, *The Physiology of Sexist and Racist Oppression, Studies in Feminist Philosophy* (Oxford; New York: Oxford University Press, 2015).

50. Christine Dunkel Schetter and Lynlee Tanner, "Anxiety, Depression and Stress in Pregnancy: Implications for Mothers, Children, Research, and Practice," *Current Opinion in Psychiatry* 25, no. 2 (March 2012): 141–48, https://doi.org/10.1097/YCO.0b013e3283503680.

51. Payscale, "The State of the Gender Pay Gap in 2021," Payscale—Salary Comparison, Salary Survey, Search Wages, n.d., https://www.payscale.com/research-and-insights/gender-pay-gap/.

52. Elise Gould, Janelle Jones, and Zane Mokhiber, "Black Workers Have Made No Progress in Closing Earnings Gaps with White Men since 2000," Economic Policy Institute (blog), September 12, 2018, https://www.epi.org/blog/black-workers-have-made-no-progress-in-closing-earnings-gaps-with-white-men-since-2000/.

53. McKinsey & Company, "Women in the Workplace 2021," September 27, 2021, https://www.mckinsey.com/featured-insights/diversity-and-inclusion/women-in-the-workplace

54. American Association of University Women, "Black Women & the Pay Gap," AAUW: Empowering Women Since 1881, n.d., https://www.aauw.org/resources/article/black-women-and-the-pay-gap/.

55. Letha A. Chadiha et al., "Empowering African American Women Informal Caregivers: A Literature Synthesis and Practice Strategies," Social Work 49, no. 1 (January 2004): 97–108, https://doi.org/10.1093/sw/49.1.97.

56. Greg R. Alexander, Michael D. Kogan, and Sara Nabukera, "Racial Differences in Prenatal Care Use in the United States: Are Disparities Decreasing?," American Journal of Public Health 92, no. 12 (December 2002): 1970–75; Institute of Medicine (US) Committee on Understanding and Eliminating Racial and Ethnic Disparities in Health Care, Unequal Treatment: Confronting Racial and Ethnic Disparities in Health Care, ed. Brian D. Smedley, Adrienne Y. Stith, and Alan R. Nelson (Washington, D.C.): National Academies Press (US), 2003), http://www.ncbi.nlm.nih.gov/books/NBK220358/.

57. Sophie Beiers, Sandra Park, and Linda Morris, "Clearing the Record: How Eviction Sealing Laws Can Advance Housing Access for Women of Color," American Civil Liberties Union, January 10, 2020, https://www.aclu.org/news/racial-justice/clearing-the-record-how-eviction-sealing-laws-can-advance-housing-access-for-women-of-color/.

58. Jing Li and Judith Scott-Clayton, "Black-White Disparity in Student Loan Debt More than Triples after Graduation," Brookings (blog), October 20, 2016, https://www.brookings.edu/research/black-white-disparity-in-student-loan-debt-more-than-triples-after-graduation/.

59. Elizabeth A. Howell et al., "Association between Hospital-Level Obstetric Quality Indicators and Maternal and Neonatal Morbidity," JAMA 312, no. 15 (October 15, 2014): 1531–41, https://doi.org/10.1001/jama.2014.13381.

60. Elizabeth A. Howell et al., "Black-White Differences in Severe Maternal Morbidity and Site of Care," American Journal of Obstetrics and Gynecology 214, no. 1 (January 2016): 122.e1–122.e7, https://doi.org/10.1016/j.ajog.2015.08.019.

61. Sarah Ruiz-Grossman, "California Takes New Steps To Stop Black Women From Dying In Childbirth," *HuffPost*, October 8, 2019, https://www.huffp ost.com/entry/california-bill-black-maternal-mortality_n_5d9cd594e 4b06ddfc50f6f0e.

62. Yousof Omeish and Samantha Kiernan, "Targeting Bias to Improve Maternal Care and Outcomes for Black Women in the USA," *EClinicalMedicine 27* (October 1, 2020), https://doi.org/10.1016/j.ecl inm.2020.100568.

63. Erica Chidi and Erica P. Cahill, "Protecting Your Birth: A Guide for Black Mothers," *The New York Times*, October 22, 2020, sec. Parenting, https://www.nytimes.com/article/black-mothers-birth.html.

64. Tim Kaine, "S.4269—116th Congress (2019-2020): Mothers and Newborns Success Act," legislation, July 22, 2020, 2019/2020, https://www.congress.gov/bill/116th-congress/senate-bill/4269.

65. Erin Brantley et al., "House-Passed Build Back Better Would Bolster Public Health Infrastructure, Health Workforce | Health Affairs Forefront," November 22, 2021, https://www.healthaffairs.org/do/10.1377/forefr ont.20211121.674613/full/.

66. Martin and Montagne, "Nothing Protects Black Women From Dying in Pregnancy and Childbirth."

67. Kelsey Butler, "Kamala Harris Rolls Out Plan to Reduce High U.S. Maternal Mortality Rates," Bloomberg.Com, December 7, 2021, https://www.bloomberg.com/news/articles/2021-12-07/kamala-harris-rolls-out-plan-for-u-s-maternal-health-crisis.

68. Michael C. Lu, "Reducing Maternal Mortality in the United States," *JAMA* 320, no. 12 (September 25, 2018): 1237–38, https://doi.org/10.1001/jama.2018.11652; Elizabeth A. Howell, "Reducing Disparities in Severe Maternal Morbidity and Mortality," *Clinical Obstetrics and Gynecology* 61, no. 2 (June 2018): 387–99, https://doi.org/10.1097/GRF.000000000 0000349.

69. Omeish and Kiernan, "Targeting Bias to Improve Maternal Care and Outcomes for Black Women in the USA."

70. Julia Belluz, "Black Moms Die in Childbirth 3 Times as Often as White Moms. Except in North Carolina.," *Vox*, July 3, 2017, https://www.vox.com/health-care/2017/7/3/15886892/black-white-moms-die-childbirth-north-carolina-less.

71. "Black Mamas Matter Alliance—Advancing Black Maternal Health," Black Mamas Matter Alliance, n.d., https://blackmamasmatter.org/.

72. "Restoring Our Own Through Transformation—RESIST," https://resist.
    org/grantee/restoring-our-own-through-transformation/.
73. Laurie Zephyrin et al., "Community-Based Models to Improve Maternal
    Health Outcomes and Promote Health Equity," March 4, 2021, https://doi.
    org/10.26099/6s6k-5330.
74. Anna North, "America Is Failing Black Moms during the Pandemic," *Vox*,
    August 10, 2020, https://www.vox.com/2020/8/10/21336312/covid-19-
    pregnancy-birth-black-maternal-mortality.
75. Roeder, "America Is Failing Its Black Mothers."

Chapter 2

1. Riya Jama, "Doctors Refused to Diagnose My Chronic Illness Because
   This World Ignores Black Women's Pain," *The Black Youth Project* (blog),
   October 16, 2018, http://blackyouthproject.com/doctors-refused-to-diagn
   ose-my-chronic-illness-because-this-world-ignores-black-womens-pain/.
2. Rolf-Detlef Treede, "The International Association for the Study of Pain
   Definition of Pain: As Valid in 2018 as in 1979, but in Need of Regularly
   Updated Footnotes," *Pain Reports* 3, no. 2 (March 5, 2018): e643, https://
   doi.org/10.1097/PR9.0000000000000643.
3. Salimah H. Meghani, Eeeseung Byun, and Rollin M. Gallagher, "Time
   to Take Stock: A Meta-Analysis and Systematic Review of Analgesic
   Treatment Disparities for Pain in the United States," *Pain Medicine
   (Malden, Mass.)* 13, no. 2 (February 2012): 150–74, https://doi.org/
   10.1111/j.1526-4637.2011.01310.x; Adil A. Shah et al., "Analgesic Access
   for Acute Abdominal Pain in the Emergency Department Among Racial/
   Ethnic Minority Patients: A Nationwide Examination," *Medical Care* 53,
   no. 12 (December 2015): 1000–1009, https://doi.org/10.1097/MLR.00000
   00000000444.
4. Monika K. Goyal et al., "Racial Disparities in Clinical pain management of
   Children With Appendicitis in Emergency Departments," *JAMA Pediatrics*
   169, no. 11 (November 2015): 996–1002, https://doi.org/10.1001/jamaped
   iatrics.2015.1915
5. Lisa J. Staton et al., "When Race Matters: Disagreement in Pain Perception
   between Patients and Their Physicians in Primary Care," *Journal of the
   National Medical Association* 99, no. 5 (May 2007): 532–38.
6. Yin Paradies et al., "Racism as a Determinant of Health: A Systematic
   Review and Meta-Analysis," *PLoS ONE* 10, no. 9 (September 23,
   2015): e0138511, https://doi.org/10.1371/journal.pone.0138511.

7. Kelly M. Hoffman et al., "Racial Bias in Pain Assessment and Treatment Recommendations, and False Beliefs about Biological Differences between Blacks and Whites," *Proceedings of the National Academy of Sciences of the United States of America* 113, no. 16 (April 19, 2016): 4296–4301, https://doi.org/10.1073/pnas.1516047113; Sophie Trawalter, Kelly M. Hoffman, and Adam Waytz, "Racial Bias in Perceptions of Others' Pain," *PLOS ONE* 7, no. 11 (November 14, 2012): 1–8, https://doi.org/10.1371/journal.pone.0048546; Sophie Trawalter, Kelly M. Hoffman, and Adam Waytz, "Correction: Racial Bias in Perceptions of Others' Pain," *PLOS ONE* 11, no. 3 (March 24, 2016): e0152334, https://doi.org/10.1371/journal.pone.0152334.

8. W. Michael Byrd and Linda A. Clayton, *An American Health Dilemma* (New York: Routledge, 2000).

9. Margaret Geneva Long, *Doctoring Freedom: The Politics of African American Medical Care in Slavery and Emancipation*, John Hope Franklin Series in African American History and Culture (Chapel Hill: University of North Carolina Press, 2012).

10. Samuel A. Cartwright, "'Report on the Diseases and Physical Peculiarities of the Negro Race,'" in *Health, Disease, and Illness: Concepts in Medicine*, ed. Arthur Caplan, James J. McCartney, and Dominic A. Sisti (Georgetown University Press, 2004), 28–39

11. Herbert C. Covey, *African-American Slave Medicine: Herbal and Non-Herbal Treatments* (Lanham: Lexington Books, 2008).

12. Stephen C. Kenny, "Medical Racism's Poison Pen: The Toxic World of Dr. Henry Ramsay (1821-1856)," *The Southern Quarterly* 54, nos. 3–4 (2016): 70–96.

13. Keisha Ray, "Blog—Inefficient Clinical pain management for Black Patients Shows That There Is a Fine Line between 'Inhumane' and 'Superhuman,'" Bioethics Today, May 4, 2016, https://bioethicstoday.org/blog/inefficient-pain-management-for-black-patients-shows-that-there-is-a-fine-line-between-inhumane-and-superhuman/.

14. Trawalter, Hoffman, and Waytz, "Racial Bias in Perceptions of Others' Pain."

15. John Hoberman, *Black and Blue: The Origins and Consequences of Medical Racism* (Los Angeles: University of California Press, 2012).

16. Kelly Serafini et al., "Racism as Experienced by Physicians of Color in the Health Care Setting," *Family Medicine* 52, no. 4 (2020): 282–87, https://doi.org/10.22454/FamMed.2020.384384.

17. Hoberman, *Black and Blue: The Origins and Consequences of Medical Racism*, 66.
18. Trawalter, Hoffman, and Waytz, "Racial Bias in Perceptions of Others' Pain."
19. George M Niles, "A Therapeutic Comparison, Medicinal and Otherwise, as Between the Caucasian and Afro-American," *Southern Medical Journal*, no. 6 (1913): 128; Hoberman, *Black and Blue: The Origins and Consequences of Medical Racism*, 109.
20. Frank R. Freemon, "The Health of the American Slave Examined by Means of Union Army Medical Statistics," *Journal of the National Medical Association* 77, no. 1 (January 1985): 50.
21. Hoberman, *Black and Blue: The Origins and Consequences of Medical Racism*.
22. Matteo Forgiarini, Marcello Gallucci, and Angelo Maravita, "Racism and the Empathy for Pain on Our Skin," *Frontiers in Psychology* 2 (2011), https://www.frontiersin.org/article/10.3389/fpsyg.2011.00108.
23. Alexandra Moffett-Bateau, "Chronic Pain, and the Denial of Care for Black Women," Rewire News Group, March 4, 2014, https://rewire.news/article/2014/03/04/chronic-pain-denial-care-black-women/.
24. Leslie R. M. Hausmann et al., "Racial Disparities in the Monitoring of Patients on Chronic Opioid Therapy," *Pain* 154, no. 1 (January 2013): 46–52, https://doi.org/10.1016/j.pain.2012.07.034.
25. Lanlan Zhang et al., "Gender Biases in Estimation of Others' Pain," *Journal of Pain* 22, no. 9 (September 2021): 1048–59, https://doi.org/10.1016/j.jpain.2021.03.001.
26. Paula T. Ross, Monica L. Lypson, and Arno K. Kumagai, "Using Illness Narratives to Explore African American Perspectives of Racial Discrimination in Health Care," *Journal of Black Studies* 43, no. 5 (July 1, 2012): 530, https://doi.org/10.1177/0021934711436129.
27. Roger Chou et al., "Clinical Guidelines for the Use of Chronic Opioid Therapy in Chronic Noncancer Pain," *Journal of Pain* 10, no. 2 (February 1, 2009): 113–130.e22, https://doi.org/10.1016/j.jpain.2008.10.008.
28. Hausmann et al., "Racial Disparities in the Monitoring of Patients on Chronic Opioid Therapy."
29. Hausmann et al., 51.
30. Nancy E. Morden et al., "Racial Inequality in Prescription Opioid Receipt—Role of Individual Health Systems," *New England Journal of Medicine* 385, no. 4 (July 22, 2021): 342–51, https://doi.org/10.1056/NEJMsa2034159.

31. Jarvis DeBerry, "When You Ignore Black People's Pain You Get a Mostly White Opioid Crisis | Opinion," NOLA, November 10, 2017, https://www.nola.com/opinions/article_886a3b60-20d5-5f4d-a680-4490ee084fe7.html.

32. Damon Tweedy, *Black Man in a White Coat: A Doctor's Reflections on Race and Medicine* (New York: Picador, 2015

33. B. Kirsch et al., "Implementation of a Clinical pain management Strategy: Identifying Pain as the Fifth Vital Sign," no. 5 (2000): 49–59; Richard A. Mularski et al., "Measuring Pain as the 5th Vital Sign Does Not Improve Quality of Clinical pain management," *Journal of General Internal Medicine* 21, no. 6 (June 2006): 607–12, https://doi.org/10.1111/j.1525-1497.2006.00415.x.

34. Carmen R. Green et al., "The Unequal Burden of Pain: Confronting Racial and Ethnic Disparities in Pain," *Pain Medicine (Malden, Mass.)* 4, no. 3 (September 2003): 277–94, https://doi.org/10.1046/j.1526-4637.2003.03034.x; Carmen Reneé Green et al., "The Effect of Race in Older Adults Presenting for Chronic Clinical pain management: A Comparative Study of Black and White Americans," *Journal of Pain* 4, no. 2 (March 2003): 82–90, https://doi.org/10.1054/jpai.2003.8.

35. Astha Singhal, Yu-Yu Tien, and Renee Y. Hsia, "Racial-Ethnic Disparities in Opioid Prescriptions at Emergency Department Visits for Conditions Commonly Associated with Prescription Drug Abuse," *PLOS ONE* 11, no. 8 (August 8, 2016): e0159224, https://doi.org/10.1371/journal.pone.0159224.

36. Singhal, Tien, and Hsia, "Racial-Ethnic Disparities in Opioid Prescriptions."

37. Tweedy, *Black Man in a White Coat*, 141.

38. Ross, Lypson, and Kumagai, "Using Illness Narratives to Explore African American Perspectives of Racial Discrimination in Health Care," 530.

39. Clarence Gravlee, "How Whiteness Works: JAMA and the Refusals of White Supremacy," *Somatosphere* (blog), March 27, 2021, http://somatosphere.net/2021/how-whiteness-works.html/; Usha Lee McFarling, "Troubling Podcast Puts JAMA, the 'voice of Medicine,' under Fire for Its Mishandling of Race," *STAT* (blog), April 6, 2021, https://www.statnews.com/2021/04/06/podcast-puts-jama-under-fire-for-mishandling-of-race/; Tanner, "Journal's 'appalling' Racism Podcast, Tweet Prompt Outcry," AP NEWS, April 28, 2021, https://apnews.com/article/race-and-ethnicity-us-news-dfab22b4929d514c55a076e81ea68440.

40. Ed Livingston, "Part 3: Interview with Dr. Mitch Katz and Host Ed Livingston (Transcript)," May 5, 2021, https://static1.squarespace.com/sta tic/5d7d985bfc6bb40f1dfae872/t/6061d1425689961a044a3ac0/161702 3298545/Transcript+-+Structural+Racism+for+Doctors.pdf.

41. JAMA, "Statement from Howard Bauchner, MD, Editor in Chief JAMA and The JAMA Network Https://T.Co/A1AJNnMWB4," Tweet, @*JAMA_ current* (blog), March 4, 2021, https://twitter.com/JAMA_current/status/ 1367546743789862912.

42. AMA, "Thread: To Start, the AMA Feels JAMA's Recent Podcast on Racism Was Wrong, False and Harmful. JAMA Maintains Editorial Independence from AMA, but We Want to Be Clear: The Podcast and Tweet Promoting It Run Counter to Current AMA Values, Policies & Actions. Https://T.Co/ UVpdMihJpt," Tweet, @*AmerMedicalAssn* (blog), March 4, 2021, https:// twitter.com/AmerMedicalAssn/status/1367551058256531459.

43. JAMA Network, *Structural Racism in Medicine and Health Care*, 2021, https://www.youtube.com/watch?v=SyzZvlvoAys.

44. American Medical Association, "AMA Announces Transition in JAMA Editorial Leadership," American Medical Association, June 1, 2021, https://www.ama-assn.org/press-center/press-releases/ama-announces- transition-jama-editorial-leadership

45. Gravlee, "How Whiteness Works."

46. Nancy Krieger et al., "Medicine's Privileged Gatekeepers: Producing Harmful Ignorance About Racism and Health | Health Affairs Forefront," April 20, 2021, https://www.healthaffairs.org/do/10.1377/forefront.20210 415.305480/full/.

47. Krieger et al., "Medicine's Privileged Gatekeepers."

48. Hardeman, R. R., Murphy, K. A., Karbeah, J., and Kozhimannil, K. B. (2018). Naming Institutionalized Racism in the Public Health Literature: A Systematic Literature Review. *Public health reports (Washington, D.C. : 1974), 133*(3), 240–249.

49. McFarling, "Troubling Podcast Puts JAMA, the 'voice of Medicine,' under Fire for Its Mishandling of Race."

50. Scott Jaschik, "Anger Over Stereotypes in Textbook," Inside Higher Ed, October 23, 2017, https://www.insidehighered.com/news/2017/10/23/ nursing-textbook-pulled-over-stereotypes

51. P. Kelley and P. Clifford, "Coping with Chronic Pain: Assessing Narrative Approaches," *Social Work* 42, no. 3 (May 1997): 266–77, https://doi.org/ 10.1093/sw/42.3.266.

52. Kosuke Kawai et al., "Adverse Impacts of Chronic Pain on Health-Related Quality of Life, Work Productivity, Depression and Anxiety in a Community-Based Study," *Family Practice* 34, no. 6 (November 16, 2017): 656–61, https://doi.org/10.1093/fampra/cmx034.

53. Lisa C. Barry et al., "Functional Self-Efficacy and Pain-Related Disability among Older Veterans with Chronic Pain in a Primary Care Setting," *Pain* 104, no. 1–2 (July 2003): 131–37, https://doi.org/10.1016/s0304-3959(02)00471-2.

54. Janiece L. Walker et al., "The Relationship between Pain, Disability and Gender in African Americans," *Clinical pain management Nursing: Official Journal of the American Society of Clinical pain management Nurses* 17, no. 5 (October 2016): 294–301, https://doi.org/10.1016/j.pmn.2016.05.007; CDC, "Infographic: Adults with Disabilities: Ethnicity and Race | CDC," Centers for Disease Control and Prevention, October 25, 2019, https://www.cdc.gov/ncbddd/disabilityandhealth/materials/infographic-disabilities-ethnicity-race.html.

55. Institute of Medicine (US) Committee on Advancing Pain Research, Care, and Education, *Relieving Pain in America: A Blueprint for Transforming Prevention, Care, Education, and Research*, The National Academies Collection: Reports Funded by National Institutes of Health (Washington, D.C.: National Academies Press, 2011), http://www.ncbi.nlm.nih.gov/books/NBK91497/.

56. Harald Breivik, Silje Endresen Reme, and Steven J. Linton, "High Risk of Depression and Suicide Attempt among Chronic Pain Patients: Always Explore Catastrophizing and Suicide Thoughts When Evaluating Chronic Pain Patients," *Scandinavian Journal of Pain* 5, no. 1 (January 1, 2014): 1–3, https://doi.org/10.1016/j.sjpain.2013.11.004.

57. Harald Breivik, Silje Endresen Reme, and Steven J. Linton, "High Risk of Depression and Suicide Attempt among Chronic Pain Patients: Always Explore Catastrophizing and Suicide Thoughts When Evaluating Chronic Pain Patients," *Scandinavian Journal of Pain* 5, no. 1 (January 1, 2014): 1–3, https://doi.org/10.1016/j.sjpain.2013.11.004.

58. CDC, "Hospitalization and Death by Race/Ethnicity," Centers for Disease Control and Prevention, March 10, 2022, https://www.cdc.gov/coronavirus/2019-ncov/covid-data/investigations-discovery/hospitalization-death-by-race-ethnicity.html.

59. Elizabeth Arias, Betzaida Tejada-Vera, and Farida Ahmed, "Provisional Life Expectancy Estimates for January through June, 2020," *National Center for Health Statistics*, Vital Statistics Rapid Release, no. 10 (2021): 8.

60. Theresa Andrasfay and Noreen Goldman, "Reductions in 2020 US Life Expectancy Due to COVID-19 and the Disproportionate Impact on the Black and Latino Populations," *Proceedings of the National Academy of Sciences* 118, no. 5 (February 2, 2021): e2014746118, https://doi.org/10.1073/pnas.2014746118.

Chapter 3

1. Mandalit del Barco and Colin Dwyer, "John Singleton, Pioneering Director Of 'Boyz N The Hood,' Dies At 51," *NPR*, April 29, 2019, sec. Movies, https://www.npr.org/2019/04/29/718219541/john-singleton-pioneering-director-of-boyz-n-the-hood-dies-at-51.
2. "John Singleton," IMDb, accessed March 19, 2022, http://www.imdb.com/name/nm0005436/awards.
3. American Heart Association News, "John Singleton's Fatal Stroke Spotlights Black Americans' Hypertension Risk," www.heart.org, May 19, 2019, https://www.heart.org/en/news/2019/05/01/john-singletons-fatal-stroke-spotlights-black-americans-hypertension-risk.
4. Milloy, "John Singleton's Death Is Another Warning Sign for Black Men. It's Time We Listen."
5. CDC, "Cardiovascular disease Facts," Centers for Disease Control and Prevention, February 7, 2022, https://www.cdc.gov/heartdisease/facts.htm.
6. Jen Thomas, "Facts and Statistics on Cardiovascular disease," Healthline, July 16, 2020, https://www.healthline.com/health/heart-disease/statistics.
7. "African Americans and Cardiovascular Disease," *The Heart Foundation* (blog), September 7, 2018, https://theheartfoundation.org/2018/09/07/african-americans-and-heart-disease/.
8. U.S. Department of Health and Human Services Office of Minority Health, "Cardiovascular Disease and African Americans," U.S. Department of Health and Human Services Office of Minority Health, January 31, 2022, https://minorityhealth.hhs.gov/omh/browse.aspx?lvl=4&lvlid=19.
9. Garth Graham, "Disparities in Cardiovascular Disease Risk in the United States," *Current Cardiology Reviews* 11, no. 3 (August 2015): 238–45, https://doi.org/10.2174/1573403X11666141122220003.
10. Salim S. Virani et al., "Cardiovascular disease and Stroke Statistics," *Circulation* 143, no. 8 (February 23, 2021): e254–743, https://doi.org/10.1161/CIR.0000000000000950.
11. American Heart Association News, "African Americans and Cardiovascular disease, Stroke," www.heart.org, July 31, 2015, https://

www.heart.org/en/health-topics/consumer-healthcare/what-is-cardiov
ascular-disease/african-americans-and-heart-disease-stroke.

12. CDC, "COVID-19 and Your Health," Centers for Disease Control and
Prevention, February 25, 2022, https://www.cdc.gov/coronavirus/2019-
ncov/need-extra-precautions/people-with-medical-conditions.html.

13. George A. Mensah, "Cardiovascular Diseases in African
Americans: Fostering Community Partnerships to Stem the Tide,"
*American Journal of Kidney Diseases: The Official Journal of the National
Kidney Foundation* 72, no. 5 Suppl 1 (November 2018): S37–42, https://doi.
org/10.1053/j.ajkd.2018.06.026; Oluwaseun Akinseye, "Cardiovascular
disease in African Americans: Why It Is More Common and What You
Can Do to Prevent It," Your Health By Methodist Le Bonheur Healthcare,
February 22, 2021, https://yourhealth.methodisthealth.org/blog/heart-
disease-in-african-americans-why-it-is-more-common-and-what-you-
can-do-to-prevent-it.

14. Stacey Jolly et al., "Higher Cardiovascular Disease Prevalence and
Mortality among Younger Blacks Compared to Whites," *American Journal
of Medicine* 123, no. 9 (September 1, 2010): 811–18, https://doi.org/
10.1016/j.amjmed.2010.04.020.

15. LaPrincess C. Brewer and Lisa A. Cooper, "Race, Discrimination,
and Cardiovascular Disease," *AMA Journal of Ethics* 16, no. 6
(June 1, 2014): 455–60, https://doi.org/10.1001/virtualmen
tor.2014.16.6.stas2-1406.

16. Graham, "Disparities in Cardiovascular Disease Risk in the United States."

17. Diane Daniel, "A Stroke at 37 Meant Relearning Everything," www.heart.
org, September 17, 2020, https://www.heart.org/en/news/2020/09/17/a-
stroke-at-37-meant-relearning-everything.

18. CDC, "Infrographic—Racial and Ethnic Disparities in Cardiovascular
disease," Health, United States Spotlight, May 2019; American Diabetes
Association, "Statistics About Diabetes | ADA," April 2, 2022, https://
www.diabetes.org/about-us/statistics/about-diabetes.

19. CDCMMWR, "QuickStats: Age-Adjusted Death Rates from Diabetes
Mellitus as Underlying or Contributing Cause Among Adults Aged ≥65
Years, by Race/Ethnicity—National Vital Statistics System, United States,
2004–2017," *Morbidity and Mortality Weekly Report* 68 (2019), https://doi.
org/10.15585/mmwr.mm6824a6; Kaiser Family Foundation, "Number of
Diabetes Deaths per 100,000 Population by Race/Ethnicity," *KFF* (blog),
March 16, 2021, https://www.kff.org/other/state-indicator/diabetes-
death-rate-by-raceethnicity/.

20. Cheryl Rucker-Whitaker, Joe Feinglass, and William H. Pearce, "Explaining Racial Variation in Lower Extremity Amputation: A 5-Year Retrospective Claims Data and Medical Record Review at an Urban Teaching Hospital," *Archives of Surgery* 138, no. 12 (December 1, 2003): 1347–51, https://doi.org/10.1001/archsurg.138.12.1347; Lizzie Presser, "The Black American Amputation Epidemic," ProPublica, May 19, 2020, https://features.propublica.org/diabetes-amputations/black-american-amputation-epidemic/.

21. John Elflein, "Physical Inactivity Prevalence by Ethnicity U.S. 2020," Statista, February 17, 2022, https://www.statista.com/statistics/252063/us-sedentary-lifestyle-among-adults-by-ethnicity/.

22. American Lung Association, "Tobacco Use in Racial and Ethnic Populations," October 14, 2020, https://www.lung.org/quit-smoking/smoking-facts/impact-of-tobacco-use/tobacco-use-racial-and-ethnic.

23. Salim S. Virani et al., "Cardiovascular disease and Stroke Statistics—2020 Update: A Report From the American Heart Association," *Circulation* 141, no. 9 (March 3, 2020), https://doi.org/10.1161/CIR.0000000000000757.

24. Vanessa Hayford, "The Humble History of Soul Food," Black Foodie, January 22, 2018, https://www.blackfoodie.co/the-humble-history-of-soul-food/.

25. African American Registry, "'Soul Food' in America, a Story (1492)," African American Registry, accessed March 19, 2022, https://aaregistry.org/story/soul-food-a-brief-history/.

26. J. M. Flack et al., "Unmasking Racial/Ethnic Disparities in Cardiovascular Disease: Nutritional, Socioeconomic, Cultural, and Health-Care-Related Contributions," in *Cardiovascular Disease in Racial and Ethnic Minorities*, ed. Keith C. Ferdinand and Annemarie Armani (Totowa, NJ: Humana Press, 2010), 51–79, https://doi.org/10.1007/978-1-59745-410-0_3.

27. U.S. Bureau of Labor Statistics, "4.9 Percent of Workers Held More than One Job at the Same Time in 2017," U.S. Department of Labor, July 19, 2018, https://www.bls.gov/opub/ted/2018/4-point-9-percent-of-workers-held-more-than-one-job-at-the-same-time-in-2017.htm.

28. Lydia Blanco, "How's Your Heart, Sis? The Alarming Truth about Black Women and Cardiovascular disease," *Black Enterprise* (blog), March 16, 2019, https://www.blackenterprise.com/hows-your-heart-sis/.

29. CDC, "Family Health History of Cardiovascular disease | CDC," Centers for Disease Control and Prevention, February 10, 2022, https://www.cdc.gov/genomics/disease/fh/history_heart_disease.htm.

30. CDC, "Know Your Risk for Cardiovascular disease," Centers for Disease Control and Prevention, December 9, 2019, https://www.cdc.gov/heart disease/risk_factors.htm.

31. Heidi L. Lujan and Stephen E. DiCarlo, "The 'African Gene' Theory: It Is Time to Stop Teaching and Promoting the Slavery Hypertension Hypothesis," *Advances in Physiology Education* 42, no. 3 (September 2018): 412–16, https://doi.org/10.1152/advan.00070.2018.

32. CardioSmart News, "Living in a Poor Neighborhood Increases Heart Failure Risk," CardioSmart—American College of Cardiology, January 22, 2018, http://www.cardiosmart.org/news/2018/1/living-in-a-poor-neigh borhood-increases-heart-failure-risk.

33. Richard Reeves, Edward Rodrigue, and Elizabeth Kneebone, "Five Evils: Multidimensional Poverty and Race in America" (The Brookings Institution, April 14, 2016).

34. Lianne Tomfohr et al., "Racial Differences in Sleep Architecture: The Role of Ethnic Discrimination," *Biological Psychology* 89, no. 1 (January 2012): 34–38, https://doi.org/10.1016/j.biopsycho.2011.09.002.

35. John H. Kingsbury, Orfeu M. Buxton, and Karen M. Emmons, "Sleep and Its Relationship to Racial and Ethnic Disparities in Cardiovascular Disease," *Current Cardiovascular Risk Reports* 7, no. 5 (October 2013): 10.1007/s12170-013-0330-0, https://doi.org/10.1007/s12170-013-0330-0; Chandra L. Jackson, Susan Redline, and Karen M. Emmons, "Sleep as a Potential Fundamental Contributor to Disparities in Cardiovascular Health," *Annual Review of Public Health* 36 (March 18, 2015): 417–40, https://doi.org/10.1146/annurev-publhealth-031914-122838.

36. American Heart Association News, "Differences Remain in Heart Attack Treatments for Black Patients," www.heart.org, September 20, 2018, https://www.heart.org/en/news/2018/09/20/differences-rem ain-in-heart-attack-treatments-for-black-patients; Sameer Arora et al., "Fifteen-Year Trends in Management and Outcomes of Non–ST-Segment–Elevation Myocardial Infarction Among Black and White Patients: The ARIC Community Surveillance Study, 2000–2014," *Journal of the American Heart Association* 7, no. 19 (October 2, 2018): e010203, https://doi.org/10.1161/JAHA.118.010203.

37. Brewer and Cooper, "Race, Discrimination, and Cardiovascular Disease."

38. Nicole Lurie et al., "Racial and Ethnic Disparities in Care: The Perspectives of Cardiologists," *Circulation* 111, no. 10 (March 15, 2005): 1264–69, https://doi.org/10.1161/01.CIR.0000157738.12783.71.

39. Matthew A. Cavender et al., "Relationship of Race/Ethnicity with Door-to-Balloon Time and Mortality in Patients Undergoing Primary Percutaneous Coronary Intervention for ST-Elevation Myocardial Infarction: Findings from Get With the Guidelines-Coronary Artery Disease," *Clinical Cardiology* 36, no. 12 (December 2013): 749–56, https://doi.org/10.1002/clc.22213.

40. Rosie Calvin et al., "Racism and Cardiovascular Disease in African Americans," *American Journal of the Medical Sciences* 325, no. 6 (June 2003): 315–31, https://doi.org/10.1097/00000441-200306000-00003.

41. Rosie Calvin et al., "Racism and Cardiovascular Disease in African Americans,"

42. Suzanne Marta, "Doctor Asked, 'Did You Know You Had a Heart Attack?,'" www.heart.org, April 23, 2021, https://www.heart.org/en/news/2021/04/23/doctor-asked-did-you-know-you-had-a-heart-attack.

43. American Heart Association News, "Cardiovascular disease in African American Women," accessed March 21, 2022, https://www.goredforwomen.org/en/about-heart-disease-in-women/facts/heart-disease-in-african-american-women.

44. Anika L. Hines and Roland J. Thorpe, "Abstract 002: Racial Disparities in Hypertension Among Young, Black and White Women, 1999-2014 National Health and Nutrition Examination Surveys," *Hypertension* 74, no. Suppl_1 (September 2019): A002–A002, https://doi.org/10.1161/hyp.74.suppl_1.002.

45. Willie M. Abel, Telisa Spikes, and Danice B. Greer, "A Qualitative Study: Hypertension Stigma Among Black Women," *Journal of Cardiovascular Nursing* 36, no. 2 (April 2021): 96–103, https://doi.org/10.1097/JCN.0000000000000759; Virani et al., "Cardiovascular disease and Stroke Statistics."

46. U.S. Department of Health and Human Services Office of Minority Health, "Cardiovascular disease and African Americans"; CDC, "Cardiovascular disease Facts."

47. Diane Daniel, "The Night before a Big Presentation, Lawyer-Mother Has a Heart Attack," www.heart.org, February 2, 2021, https://www.heart.org/en/news/2021/02/02/the-night-before-a-big-presentation-lawyer-mother-has-a-heart-attack.

48. Evette Dionne, "What No One Tells Black Women About Cardiovascular disease," *ZORA* (blog), May 21, 2020, https://zora.medium.com/what-no-one-tells-black-women-about-heart-disease-af2c037eeae3.

49. Harry J. Holzer, "Why Are Employment Rates so Low among Black Men?," *Brookings* (blog), March 1, 2021, https://www.brookings.edu/research/why-are-employment-rates-so-low-among-black-men/.

50. American Heart Association, "Heart Attack Symptoms in Women," www.heart.org, July 31, 2015, https://www.heart.org/en/health-topics/heart-att ack/warning-signs-of-a-heart-attack/heart-attack-symptoms-in-women.

51. Kevin A. Schulman et al., "The Effect of Race and Sex on Physicians' Recommendations for Cardiac Catheterization," *New England Journal of Medicine* 340, no. 8 (February 25, 1999): 618–26, https://doi.org/10.1056/NEJM199902253400806.

52. NEJM Group, "Racial Disparities in Clinical Medicine: Conversations, Perspectives, and Research on Advancing Medical Equity" (Massachusetts Medical Society, 2021), https://store.nejm.org/media/assets/nejm/regis ter/pdf/NEJM_Group_Racial_Disparities_in_Clinical_Medicine.pdf.

53. Virani et al., "Cardiovascular disease and Stroke Statistics."

54. CDC, "A Closer Look at African American Men and High Blood Pressure Control: A Review of Psychosocial Factors and Systems-Level Interventions" (Centers for Disease Control and Prevention, 2010).

55. Lisandro D. Colantonio et al., "Black-White Differences in Incident Fatal, Nonfatal and Total Coronary Cardiovascular disease," *Circulation* 136, no. 2 (July 11, 2017): 152–66, https://doi.org/10.1161/CIRCULATION AHA.116.025848.

56. Arch G. Mainous et al., "Trends in Cardiovascular Disease Risk in the U.S., 1999–2014," *American Journal of Preventive Medicine* 55, no. 3 (September 1, 2018): 384–88, https://doi.org/10.1016/j.amepre.2018.04.025.

57. Wizdom Powell Hammond, Derrick Matthews, and Giselle Corbie-Smith, "Psychosocial Factors Associated With Routine Health Examination Scheduling and Receipt Among African American Men," *Journal of the National Medical Association* 102, no. 4 (April 1, 2010): 276–89, https://doi.org/10.1016/S0027-9684(15)30600-3.

58. Elise Gould, Janelle Jones, and Zane Mokhiber, "Black Workers Have Made No Progress in Closing Earnings Gaps with White Men since 2000," *Economic Policy Institute* (blog), September 12, 2018, https://www.epi.org/blog/black-workers-have-made-no-progress-in-closing-earnings-gaps-with-white-men-since-2000/.

59. Jackson Gruver, "Racial Wage Gap for Men," Payscale—Salary Comparison, Salary Survey, Search Wages, May 7, 2019, https://www.payscale.com/research-and-insights/racial-wage-gap-for-men/.

60. Holzer, "Why Are Employment Rates so Low among Black Men?"

61. Katharina Buchholz, "Infographic: Black Incarceration Rates Are Dropping in the U.S.," Statista Infographics, February 19, 2021, https://www.statista.com/chart/18376/us-incarceration-rates-by-sex-and-race-ethnic-origin/.

62. Rodolfo A. Bulatao, Norman B. Anderson, and Ethnicity National Research Council (US) Panel on Race, Stress, *Understanding Racial and Ethnic Differences in Health in Late Life: A Research Agenda* (National Academies Press (US), 2004), https://www.ncbi.nlm.nih.gov/books/NBK24685/.

63. CDC, "A Closer Look at African American Men and High Blood Pressure Control: A Review of Psychosocial Factors and Systems-Level Interventions."

64. A. Rozanski, J. A. Blumenthal, and J. Kaplan, "Impact of Psychological Factors on the Pathogenesis of Cardiovascular Disease and Implications for Therapy," *Circulation* 99, no. 16 (April 27, 1999): 2192–2217, https://doi.org/10.1161/01.cir.99.16.2192.

65. Dorothy D. Dunlop et al., "Racial/Ethnic Differences in Rates of Depression among Preretirement Adults," *American Journal of Public Health* 93, no. 11 (November 2003): 1945–52, https://doi.org/10.2105/ajph.93.11.1945.

66. Stephanie Reaves, "Mental Health Association in Delaware," *Minority Mental Health Month* (blog), July 5, 2021, https://www.mhainde.org/minority-mental-health-month/.

67. Somnath Saha and Mary Catherine Beach, "Impact of Physician Race on Patient Decision-Making and Ratings of Physicians: A Randomized Experiment Using Video Vignettes," *Journal of General Internal Medicine* 35, no. 4 (April 1, 2020): 1084–91, https://doi.org/10.1007/s11606-020-05646-z.

68. Erin C. Strumpf, "Racial/Ethnic Disparities in Primary Care: The Role of Physician-Patient Concordance," *Medical Care* 49, no. 5 (May 2011): 496–503, https://doi.org/10.1097/MLR.0b013e31820fbee4.

69. Ana H. Traylor et al., "Adherence to Cardiovascular Disease Medications: Does Patient-Provider Race/Ethnicity and Language Concordance Matter?," *Journal of General Internal Medicine* 25, no. 11 (November 2010): 1172–77, https://doi.org/10.1007/s11606-010-1424-8.

70. Nao Hagiwara et al., "Physician Racial Bias and Word Use during Racially Discordant Medical Interactions," *Health Communication* 32, no. 4 (April 2017): 401–8, https://doi.org/10.1080/10410236.2016.1138389.

71. Marcella Alsan, Owen Garrick, and Grant C. Graziani, "Does Diversity Matter for Health? Experimental Evidence from Oakland," Working Paper, Working Paper Series (National Bureau of Economic Research, June 2018), https://doi.org/10.3386/w24787.

72. Hagiwara et al., "Physician Racial Bias and Word Use during Racially Discordant Medical Interactions."

73. AAMC Staff, "Figure 18. Percentage of All Active Physicians by Race/ Ethnicity, 2018," AAMC—Association of American Medical Colleges, 2019, https://www.aamc.org/data-reports/workforce/interactive-data/fig ure-18-percentage-all-active-physicians-race/ethnicity-2018.

74. Lauren A. Taylor et al., "Should a Healthcare System Facilitate Racially Concordant Care for Black Patients?," *Pediatrics* 148, no. 4 (October 1, 2021): e2021051113, https://doi.org/10.1542/peds.2021-051113.

75. Keith Churchwell et al., "Call to Action: Structural Racism as a Fundamental Driver of Health Disparities: A Presidential Advisory From the American Heart Association," *Circulation* 142, no. 24 (December 15, 2020): e454–68, https://doi.org/10.1161/CIR.0000000000000936.

76. Lesli E. Skolarus et al., "Considerations in Addressing Social Determinants of Health to Reduce Racial/Ethnic Disparities in Stroke Outcomes in the United States," *Stroke* 51, no. 11 (November 2020): 3433–39, https://doi. org/10.1161/STROKEAHA.120.030426.

77. Jonathan Kahn, *Race in a Bottle: The Story of BiDil and Racialized Medicine in a Post-Genomic Age* (Columbia University Press, 2012).

Chapter 4

1. Brian Resnick, "The Racial Inequality of Sleep," *The Atlantic*, October 27, 2015, https://www.theatlantic.com/health/archive/2015/10/the-sleep-gap-and-racial-inequality/412405/.

2. Kirsten Nunez and Karen Lamoreux, "Why Do We Sleep?," *Healthline*, July 20, 2020, https://www.healthline.com/health/why-do-we-sleep.

3. CDC, "Sleep and Sleep Disorders," Centers for Disease Control and Prevention, April 15, 2020, https://www.cdc.gov/sleep/index.html.

4. Eric Suni, "Sleep Disorders and Race: What's the Connection?," Sleep Foundation, November 4, 2017, https://www.sleepfoundation.org/how-sleep-works/whats-connection-between-race-and-sleep-disorders; Joao Nunes et al., "Sleep Duration among Black and White Americans: Results of the National Health Interview Survey," *Journal of the National Medical Association* 100, no. 3 (March 2008): 317–22, https://doi.org/10.1016/

s0027-9684(15)31244-x; Nirav P. Patel et al., "'Sleep Disparity' in the Population: Poor Sleep Quality Is Strongly Associated with Poverty and Ethnicity," *BMC Public Health* 10, no. 1 (August 11, 2010): 475, https://doi.org/10.1186/1471-2458-10-475; Megan E. Ruiter et al., "Normal Sleep in African-Americans and Caucasian-Americans: A Meta-Analysis," *Sleep Medicine* 12, no. 3 (March 2011): 209–14, https://doi.org/10.1016/j.sleep.2010.12.010; Chandra L. Jackson et al., "Racial Disparities in Short Sleep Duration by Occupation and Industry," *American Journal of Epidemiology* 178, no. 9 (November 1, 2013): 1442–51, https://doi.org/10.1093/aje/kwt159.

5. Elizabeth J. Mezick et al., "Influence of Race and Socioeconomic Status on Sleep: Pittsburgh Sleep SCORE Project," *Psychosomatic Medicine* 70, no. 4 (May 2008): 410–16, https://doi.org/10.1097/PSY.0b013e31816fdf21.

6. Diane S. Lauderdale et al., "Objectively Measured Sleep Characteristics among Early-Middle-Aged Adults: The CARDIA Study," *American Journal of Epidemiology* 164, no. 1 (July 1, 2006): 5–16, https://doi.org/10.1093/aje/kwj199.

7. Michael A. Grandner et al., "Sleep Disparity, Race/Ethnicity, and Socioeconomic Position," *Sleep Medicine* 18 (February 2016): 7–18, https://doi.org/10.1016/j.sleep.2015.01.020; John H. Kingsbury, Orfeu M. Buxton, and Karen M. Emmons, "Sleep and Its Relationship to Racial and Ethnic Disparities in Cardiovascular Disease," *Current Cardiovascular Risk Reports* 7, no. 5 (October 2013): 10.1007/s12170-013-0330-0, https://doi.org/10.1007/s12170-013-0330-0; Jackson et al., "Racial Disparities in Short Sleep Duration by Occupation and Industry."

8. Elizabeth Arias, Betzaida Tejada-Vera, and Farida Ahmed, "Provisional Life Expectancy Estimates for January through June, 2020," *National Center for Health Statistics*, Vital Statistics Rapid Release, no. 10 (2021): 8.

9. David Leonhardt, "Middle-Class Black Families, in Low-Income Neighborhoods," *The New York Times*, June 24, 2015, sec. The Upshot, https://www.nytimes.com/2015/06/25/upshot/middle-class-black-famil ies-in-low-income-neighborhoods.html.

10. Lauren Hale and Benjamin Hale, "Treat the Source Not the Symptoms: Why Thinking about Sleep Informs the Social Determinants of Health," *Health Education Research* 25, no. 3 (June 2010): 395–400, https://doi.org/10.1093/her/cyq027.

11. Lauren Hale et al., "Perceived Neighborhood Quality, Sleep Quality, and Health Status: Evidence from the Survey of the Health of Wisconsin,"

Social Science & Medicine (1982) 79 (February 2013): 16–22, https://doi. org/10.1016/j.socscimed.2012.07.021.

12. Hale et al.

13. Resnick, "The Racial Inequality of Sleep."

14. Richard Rothstein, *The Color of Law: A Forgotten History of How Our Government Segregated America,* First edition (New York; London: Liveright Publishing Corporation, a division of W. W. Norton & Company, 2017); Keisha Ray, "Black and Sleepless in a Nonideal World," in *Applying Nonideal Theory to Bioethics: Living and Dying in a Nonideal World,* ed. Elizabeth Victor and Laura K. Guidry-Grimes (Springer, 2021), 235–54.

15. Rothstein, *The Color of Law*; Ray, "Black and Sleepless in a Nonideal World."

16. Cecilia Rouse et al., "Exclusionary Zoning: Its Effect on Racial Discrimination in the Housing Market," The White House, June 17, 2021, https://www.whitehouse.gov/cea/written-materials/2021/06/17/exclu sionary-zoning-its-effect-on-racial-discrimination-in-the-housing- market/.

17. Equitable Housing Institute, "Exclusionary Housing Policies," EHI— Equitable Housing Institute, accessed April 25, 2019, https://www.equit ablehousing.org/background/exclusionary-housing-practices/198-exclu sionary-housing-practices.html; Sharon Perlman Krefetz, "Low- and Moderate-Income Housing in the Suburbs: The Massachusetts 'Anti-Snob Zoning' Law Experience," *Policy Studies Journal* 8, no. 2 (1979): 288–99, https://doi.org/10.1111/j.1541-0072.1979.tb01580.x.

18. Rouse et al., "Exclusionary Zoning."

19. U.S. Department of and Housing and Urban Development, "History of Fair Housing," U.S. Department of Housing and Urban Development (HUD), accessed June 9, 2020, https://www.hud.gov/program_offices/fai r_housing_equal_opp/aboutfheo/history.

20. Rothstein, *The Color of Law*; Ray, "Black and Sleepless in a Nonideal World."

21. Keeanga-Yamahtta Taylor, *Race for Profit: How Banks and the Real Estate Industry Undermined Black Homeownership,* (Chapel Hill; University of North Carolina Press, 2019)

22. Alanna McCargo, "A Five-Point Strategy for Reducing the Black Homeownership Gap," Urban Institute, February 14, 2019, https://www. urban.org/urban-wire/five-point-strategy-reducing-black-homeowners hip-gap.

23. Emmanuel Martinez and Lauren Kirchner, "The Secret Bias Hidden in Mortgage-Approval Algorithms," The Markup, August 25, 2021, https://themarkup.org/denied/2021/08/25/the-secret-bias-hidden-in-mortgage-approval-algorithms.

24. Richard Reeves et al., "Five Evils: Multidimensional Poverty and Race in America," The Brookings Institution, April 2016, https://www.brookings.edu/wp-content/uploads/2016/06/reeveskneebonerodrigue_multidimensionalpoverty_fullpaper.pdf.

25. Christopher W. Tessum et al., "PM 2.5 Polluters Disproportionately and Systemically Affect People of Color in the United States," Science Advances 7 no. 18, (April 28, 2021): eabf4491, https://doi.org/10.1126/sciadv.abf4491.

26. Luke W. Cole and Sheila R. Foster, From the Ground Up: Environmental Racism and the Rise of the Environmental Justice Movement, (New York: NYU Press, 2000).

27. CDC, "Child Asthma Prevalence by Race and State/Territory," Centers for Disease Control and Prevention, June 11, 2018, https://www.cdc.gov/asthma/asthmadata/Child_Prevalence_Race.html.

28. United States Environmental Protection Agency, "Children's Environmental Health Disparities: Black and African American Children and Asthma," Overviews and Factsheets, May 20, 2014, https://www.epa.gov/children/childrens-environmental-health-disparities-black-and-african-american-children-and-asthma; U.S. Department of Health and Human Services Office of Minority Health, "Asthma and African Americans—The Office of Minority Health," U.S. Department of Health and Human Services Office of Minority Health, November 2, 2021, https://minorityhealth.hhs.gov/omh/browse.aspx?lvl=4&lvlid=15.

29. Sara E. Grineski and Timothy W. Collins, "Geographic and Social Disparities in Exposure to Air Neurotoxicants at U.S. Public Schools," Environmental Research 161 (February 2018): 580–87, https://doi.org/10.1016/j.envres.2017.11.047.

30. Lauren Zanolli, "'We're Just Waiting to Die': The Black Residents Living on Top of a Toxic Landfill Site," The Guardian, December 11, 2019, sec. US news, https://www.theguardian.com/us-news/2019/dec/11/gordon-plaza-louisiana-toxic-landfill-site; Keisha Ray, "In the Name of Racial Justice: Why Bioethics Should Care About Environmental Toxins," Hastings Center Report 51, no. 3 (2021): 23–26, https://doi.org/10.1002/hast.1251.

31. Tegan Wendland, "New Gas and Chemical Facilities Crowd Louisiana's 'Cancer Alley,'" *NPR*, March 10, 2020, sec. Environment, https://www.npr.org/2020/03/10/813922168/new-gas-and-chemical-facilities-crowd-lou isianas-cancer-alley.

32. Tristan Baurick, Lylla Younes, and Joan Meiners, "Polluter's Paradise: Welcome to 'Cancer Alley,' Where Toxic Air Is About to Get Worse," ProPublica, October 30, 2019, https://www.propublica.org/article/welcome-to-cancer-alley-where-toxic-air-is-about-to-get-worse?token=PfkMUk0VOJFLCI7ofscfo7VgS3x9ll1i.

33. Jamiles Lartey and Oliver Laughland, "'Almost Every Household Has Someone That Has Died from Cancer,'" The Guardian, 20119-05-06, http://www.theguardian.com/us-news/ng-interactive/2019/may/06/can certown-louisana-reserve-special-report.

34. Erin Douglas, "Cancer Cluster Identified in Neighborhood near Union Pacific Rail Yard's Contamination," Houston Chronicle, December 6, 2019, https://www.houstonchronicle.com/business/article/Cancer-clus ter-identified-in-Houston-neighborhood-14885972.php.

35. Garth N. Graham, "Why Your ZIP Code Matters More Than Your Genetic Code: Promoting Healthy Outcomes from Mother to Child," *Breastfeeding Medicine* 11, no. 8 (October 2016): 396–97, https://doi.org/10.1089/bfm.2016.0113.

36. Sanne Magnan, "Social Determinants of Health 101 for Health Care: Five Plus Five," *NAM Perspectives*, October 9, 2017, https://doi.org/10.31478/201710c; Emily Orminski, "Your Zip Code Is More Important than Your Genetic Code," NCRC," June 30, 2021, https://www.ncrc.org/your-zip-code-is-more-important-than-your-genetic-code/.

37. Oladipupo Olafiranye et al., "Obstructive Sleep Apnea and Cardiovascular Disease in Blacks: A Call to Action from Association of Black Cardiologists," *American Heart Journal* 165, no. 4 (April 2013): 468–76, https://doi.org/10.1016/j.ahj.2012.12.018.

38. Margaret T. Hicken et al., "'Every Shut Eye, Ain't Sleep': The Role of Racism-Related Vigilance in Racial/Ethnic Disparities in Sleep Difficulty," *Race and Social Problems* 5, no. 2 (June 1, 2013): 100–112, https://doi.org/10.1007/s12552-013-9095-9.

39. Lianne Tomfohr et al., "Racial Differences in Sleep Architecture: The Role of Ethnic Discrimination," *Biological Psychology* 89, no. 1 (January 2012): 34–38, https://doi.org/10.1016/j.biopsycho.2011.09.002.

40. Hicken et al., "'Every Shut Eye, Ain't Sleep.'"

41. Hicken et al., 102.

42. Amir Vera and Laura Ly, "White Woman Who Called Police on a Black Man Bird-Watching in Central Park Has Been Fired," CNN, May 26, 2020, https://www.cnn.com/2020/05/26/us/central-park-video-dog-video-afri can-american-trnd/index.html.

43. Tommy J. Curry, *The Man-Not: Race, Class, Genre, and the Dilemmas of Black Manhood* (Philadelphia: Temple University Press, 2017).

44. Nicholas Kristof, "What If There Were No George Floyd Video?," *The New York Times*, June 6, 2020, sec. Opinion, https://www.nytimes.com/ 2020/06/06/opinion/sunday/george-floyd-structural-racism.html.

45. Hicken et al., " 'Every Shut Eye, Ain't Sleep,' " 102.

46. Hale and Hale, "Treat the Source Not the Symptoms."

47. Hicken et al., " 'Every Shut Eye, Ain't Sleep.' "

48. Hicken et al.

49. Douglas Quenqua, "How Well You Sleep May Hinge on Race," *The New York Times*, August 20, 2012, sec. Health, https://www.nytimes.com/ 2012/08/21/health/how-well-you-sleep-may-hinge-on-race.html.

50. Tomfohr et al., "Racial Differences in Sleep Architecture."

51. Suni, "Sleep Hygiene," Sleep Foundation, November 29, 2021, https:// www.sleepfoundation.org/sleep-hygiene.

52. CDC, "Tips for Better Sleep," Centers for Disease Control and Prevention, July 15, 2016, https://www.cdc.gov/sleep/about_sleep/sleep_hygi ene.html.

53. Ray, "Black and Sleepless in a Nonideal World."

54. Charles W. Mills, "'Ideal Theory' as Ideology," *Hypatia* 20, no. 3 (2005): 172, https://doi.org/10.1353/hyp.2005.0107.

55. Grandner et al., "Sleep Disparity, Race/Ethnicity, and Socioeconomic Position."

56. Jonathan Kaplan, "Self-Care as Self Blame Redux: Stress as Personal and Political," *Kennedy Institute of Ethics Journal* 29, no. 2 (June 2019): 97–123

References

American Medical Association. 2021. "Advancing Health Equity: A Guide to Language, Narrative and Concepts." https://www.ama-assn.org/system/files/ama-aamc-equity-guide.pdf.

"Black Mamas Matter Alliance—Advancing Black Maternal Health." n.d. *Black Mamas Matter Alliance.* https://blackmamasmatter.org/.

"Encyclopedia of Social Problems." 2022. In *One Drop Rule.* Los Angeles, Sage Publishing, https://us.sagepub.com/en-us/nam/encyclopedia-of-social-problems/book229800.

"Fact Sheet: The State of African American Women in the United States." n.d. *Center for American Progress (blog).* https://www.americanprogress.org/article/fact-sheet-the-state-of-african-american-women-in-the-united-states/.

"Maternal Mortality Rates in the United States, 2020," CDC, February 23, 2022, https://www.cdc.gov/nchs/data/hestat/maternal-mortality/2020/maternal-mortality-rates-2020.htm.

"Restoring Our Own Through Transformation—RESIST." n.d. Accessed February 12, 2022. https://resist.org/grantee/restoring-our-own-through-transformation/.

AAMC Staff. 2019. "Figure 18. Percentage of All Active Physicians by Race/Ethnicity, 2018." AAMC—Association of American Medical Colleges. https://www.aamc.org/data-reports/workforce/interactive-data/figure-18-percentage-all-active-physicians-race/ethnicity-2018.

Abel, Willie M., Telisa Spikes, and Danice B. Greer. 2021. "A Qualitative Study: Hypertension Stigma Among Black Women." *Journal of Cardiovascular Nursing 36,* no. 2 (April): 96–103. https://doi.org/10.1097/JCN.0000000000000759.

Adger, W. Neil. 2000. "Social and Ecological Resilience: Are They Related?" *Progress in Human Geography 24* (3): 347–64. https://doi.org/10.1191/030913200701540465.

African American Registry. 2022. "'Soul Food' in America, a Story (1492)." African American Registry. Accessed March 19. https://aaregistry.org/story/soul-food-a-brief-history/.

Akinseye, Oluwaseun A., Stephen K. Williams, Azizi Seixas, Seithikurippu R. Pandi-Perumal, Julian Vallon, Ferdinand Zizi, and Girardin Jean-Louis. 2015. "Sleep as a Mediator in the Pathway Linking Environmental Factors to Hypertension: A Review of the Literature." *International Journal of Hypertension 2015:* 926414. https://doi.org/10.1155/2015/926414.

Akinseye, Oluwaseun. 2021. "Cardiovascular disease in African Americans: Why It Is More Common and What You Can Do to Prevent It." Your Health By Methodist Le Bonheur Healthcare, February 22. https:// yourhealth.methodisthealth.org/blog/heart-disease-in-african-americans-why-it-is-more-common-and-what-you-can-do-to-prevent-it.

Alexander, Greg R., Michael D. Kogan, and Sara Nabukera. 2002. "Racial Differences in Prenatal Care Use in the United States: Are Disparities Decreasing?" *American Journal of Public Health 92* (12): 1970–75.

Almasy, Steve. 2020. "Detroit Bus Driver Jason Hargrove Dies Days after Making Video about Coughing Passenger." *CNN.* May 3, 2020. https:// www.cnn.com/2020/04/03/us/detroit-bus-driver-dies-coronavirus-trnd/index.html.

Alsan, Marcella, Owen Garrick, and Grant C. Graziani. 2018. "Does Diversity Matter for Health? Experimental Evidence from Oakland." Working Paper. Working Paper Series. National Bureau of Economic Research, June. https:// doi.org/10.3386/w24787.

AMA. 2021. "Thread: To Start, the AMA Feels JAMA's Recent Podcast on Racism Was Wrong, False and Harmful. JAMA Maintains Editorial Independence from AMA, but We Want to Be Clear: The Podcast and Tweet Promoting It Run Counter to Current AMA Values, Policies & Actions. Https://T.Co/UVpdMihJpt." Tweet. *@AmerMedicalAssn* (blog), March 4. https://twitter.com/AmerMedicalAssn/status/1367551058256531459.

American Association of University Women. n.d. "*Black Women & the Pay Gap.*" AAUW: Empowering Women Since 1881. https://www.aauw.org/resources/article/black-women-and-the-pay-gap/.

American Diabetes Association. 2022. "Statistics About Diabetes | ADA," April 2. https://www.diabetes.org/about-us/statistics/about-diabetes.

American Heart Association News. 2015. "African Americans and Cardiovascular disease, Stroke." www.heart.org, July 31. https://www.heart.org/en/health-topics/consumer-healthcare/what-is-cardiovascular-disease/african-americans-and-heart-disease-stroke.

American Heart Association News. 2018. "Differences Remain in Heart Attack Treatments for Black Patients." www.heart.org, September 20. https://www.heart.org/en/news/2018/09/20/differences-remain-in-heart-attack-treatments-for-black-patients.

American Heart Association News. 2019. "John Singleton's Fatal Stroke Spotlights Black Americans' Hypertension Risk." www.heart.org, May 19. https://www.heart.org/en/news/2019/05/01/john-singletons-fatal-stroke-spotlights-black-americans-hypertension-risk.

American Heart Association News. 2022. "Cardiovascular disease in African American Women." Accessed March 21. https://www.goredforwomen.org/en/about-heart-disease-in-women/facts/heart-disease-in-african-american-women.

American Heart Association. 2015. "Heart Attack Symptoms in Women." www.heart.org, July 31. https://www.heart.org/en/health-topics/heart-att ack/warning-signs-of-a-heart-attack/heart-attack-symptoms-in-women.

American Lung Association. 2020. "Tobacco Use in Racial and Ethnic Populations," October 14. https://www.lung.org/quit-smoking/smoking-facts/impact-of-tobacco-use/tobacco-use-racial-and-ethnic.

American Medical Association. 2021. "AMA Announces Transition in JAMA Editorial Leadership." American Medical Association, June 1. https://www.ama-assn.org/press-center/press-releases/ama-announces-transition-jama-editorial-leadership.

Andrasfay, Theresa, and Noreen Goldman. 2021. "Reductions in 2020 US Life Expectancy Due to COVID-19 and the Disproportionate Impact on the Black and Latino Populations." *Proceedings of the National Academy of Sciences 118*, no. 5 (February 2): e2014746118. https://doi.org/10.1073/pnas.2014746118.

Arias, Elizabeth, Betzaida Tejada-Vera, and Farida Ahmed. 2021. "Provisional Life Expectancy Estimates for January through June, 2020." *National Center for Health Statistics*, Vital Statistics Rapid Release, no. 10: 8.

Arora, Sameer, George A. Stouffer, Anna Kucharska-Newton, Muthiah Vaduganathan, Arman Qamar, Kunihiro Matsushita, Dhaval Kolte, et al. 2018. "Fifteen-Year Trends in Management and Outcomes of Non–ST-Segment–Elevation Myocardial Infarction Among Black and White Patients: The ARIC Community Surveillance Study, 2000–2014." *Journal of the American Heart Association 7*, no. 19 (October 2): e010203. https://doi.org/10.1161/JAHA.118.010203.

Baptiste, Edward. 2014. *The Half Has Never Been Told: Slavery and the Making of American Capitalism*. New York: Basic Books.

Barco, Mandalit del, and Colin Dwyer. 2019. "John Singleton, Pioneering Director Of 'Boyz N The Hood,' Dies At 51." *NPR*, April 29, sec. Movies. https://www.npr.org/2019/04/29/718219541/john-singleton-pioneering-director-of-boyz-n-the-hood-dies-at-51.

Barry, Lisa C., Zhenchao Guo, Robert D. Kerns, Bao D. Duong, and M. Carrington Reid. 2003. "Functional Self-Efficacy and Pain-Related Disability among Older Veterans with Chronic Pain in a Primary Care Setting." *Pain 104*, nos. 1–2 (July): 131–37. https://doi.org/10.1016/s0304-3959(02)00471-2.

Barthole, Jenn. 2022. "*Black Maternal Health Week: Serena Williams Shares Her Near-Fatal Birthing Story.*" *Ebony*. https://www.ebony.com/lifestyle/serena-williams-shares-her-near-fatal-birthing-story1/.

Baurick, Tristan, Lylla Younes, and Joan Meiners. 2019. "Polluter's Paradise: Welcome to 'Cancer Alley,' Where Toxic Air Is About to Get Worse." *ProPublica*, October 30. https://www.propublica.org/article/welcome-to-cancer-alley-where-toxic-air-is-about-to-get-worse?token=PfkMUk0VOJFLCI7ofscfo7VgS3x9ll1i.

BBC. 2018. "New York: James Marion Sims Statue Removed From Central Park." *BBC News.* https://www.bbc.com/news/world-us-canada-43804725.

Bean, Meghan G., Jeff Stone, Terry A. Badger, Elizabeth S. Focella, and Gordon B. Moskowitz. 2013. "Evidence of Nonconscious Stereotyping of Hispanic Patients by Nursing and Medical Students." *Nursing Research 62* (5): 362–67. https://doi.org/10.1097/NNR.0b013e31829e02ec.

Beiers, Sophie, Sandra Park, and Linda Morris. 2020. "Clearing the Record: How Eviction Sealing Laws Can Advance Housing Access for Women of Color." American Civil Liberties Union. January 10, 2020. https://www.aclu.org/news/racial-justice/clearing-the-record-how-evict ion-sealing-laws-can-advance-housing-access-for-women-of-color/.

Bell, Carl C., and Harshad Mehta. 1980. "The Misdiagnosis of Black Patients with Manic Depressive Illness." *Journal of the National Medical Association 72* (2): 141–45.

Belluz, Julia. 2017. "Black Moms Die in Childbirth 3 Times as Often as White Moms. Except in North Carolina." *Vox.* July 3, 2017. https://www.vox.com/ health-care/2017/7/3/15886892/black-white-moms-die-childbirth-north-carolina-less.

Blanco, Lydia. 2019. "How's Your Heart, Sis? The Alarming Truth about Black Women and Cardiovascular disease." *Black Enterprise* (blog), March 16. https://www.blackenterprise.com/hows-your-heart-sis/.

Blendon, R. J., L. H. Aiken, H. E. Freeman, and C. R. Corey. 1989. "Access to Medical Care for Black and White Americans. A Matter of Continuing Concern." *JAMA 261* (2): 278–81.

Brantley, Erin, Mandar Bodas, Candice Chen, Patricia Pittman, Jeffrey Levi, Naomi Seiler, Anne Markus, Marsha Regenstein, Peter Shin, and Sara Rosenbaum. 2021. "House-Passed Build Back Better Would Bolster Public Health Infrastructure, Health Workforce | Health Affairs Forefront." November 22, 2021. https://www.healthaffairs.org/do/10.1377/forefr ont.20211121.674613/full/.

Breivik, Harald, Silje Endresen Reme, and Steven J. Linton. 2014. "High Risk of Depression and Suicide Attempt among Chronic Pain Patients: Always Explore Catastrophizing and Suicide Thoughts When Evaluating Chronic Pain Patients." *Scandinavian Journal of Pain 5*, no. 1 (January 1): 1–3. https:// doi.org/10.1016/j.sjpain.2013.11.004.

Brewer, LaPrincess C., and Lisa A. Cooper. 2014. "Race, Discrimination, and Cardiovascular Disease." *AMA Journal of Ethics 16*, no. 6 (June 1): 455–60. https://doi.org/10.1001/virtualmentor.2014.16.6.stas2-1406.

Buchholz, Katharina. 2021. "Infographic: Black Incarceration Rates Are Dropping in the U.S." Statista Infographics, February 19. https://www. statista.com/chart/18376/us-incarceration-rates-by-sex-and-race-ethnic-origin/.

Bulatao, Rodolfo A., Norman B. Anderson, and Ethnicity National Research Council (US) Panel on Race. 2004. *Stress. Understanding Racial and Ethnic Differences in Health in Late Life: A Research Agenda*. National Academies Press (US). https://www.ncbi.nlm.nih.gov/books/NBK24685/.

Butler, Kelsey. 2021. "Kamala Harris Rolls Out Plan to Reduce High U.S. Maternal Mortality Rates." Bloomberg.Com, December 7, 2021. https://www.bloomberg.com/news/articles/2021-12-07/kamala-harris-rolls-out-plan-for-u-s-maternal-health-crisis.

Byrd, W. Michael, and Linda A. Clayton. 2000. *An American Health Dilemma*. New York: Routledge.

Calvin, Rosie, Karen Winters, Sharon B. Wyatt, David R. Williams, Frances C. Henderson, and Evelyn R. Walker. 2003. "Racism and Cardiovascular Disease in African Americans." *American Journal of the Medical Sciences* 325, no. 6 (June): 315–31. https://doi.org/10.1097/00000441-200306000-00003.

CardioSmart News. 2018. "Living in a Poor Neighborhood Increases Heart Failure Risk." CardioSmart—American College of Cardiology, January 22. http://www.cardiosmart.org/news/2018/1/living-in-a-poor-neighborhood-increases-heart-failure-risk.

Cartwright, Samuel A. 2004. "'Report on the Diseases and Physical Peculiarities of the Negro Race.'" In *Health, Disease, and Illness: Concepts in Medicine*, edited by Arthur Caplan, James J. McCartney, and Dominic A. Sisti, 28–39. Georgetown University Press.

Cavender, Matthew A., Andrew N. Rassi, Gregg C. Fonarow, Christopher P. Cannon, W. Frank Peacock, Warren K. Laskey, Adrian F. Hernandez, et al. 2013. "Relationship of Race/Ethnicity with Door-to-Balloon Time and Mortality in Patients Undergoing Primary Percutaneous Coronary Intervention for ST-Elevation Myocardial Infarction: Findings from Get With the Guidelines-Coronary Artery Disease." *Clinical Cardiology* 36, no. 12 (December): 749–56. https://doi.org/10.1002/clc.22213.

CDC. 2010. *"A Closer Look at African American Men and High Blood Pressure Control: A Review of Psychosocial Factors and Systems-Level Interventions."* Centers for Disease Control and Prevention.

CDC. 2016. "Tips for Better Sleep." Centers for Disease Control and Prevention, July 15. https://www.cdc.gov/sleep/about_sleep/sleep_hygiene.html.

CDC. 2018. "Child Asthma Prevalence by Race and State/Territory." *Centers for Disease Control and Prevention*, June 11. https://www.cdc.gov/asthma/asthmadata/Child_Prevalence_Race.html.

CDC. 2019. "Infographic: Adults with Disabilities: Ethnicity and Race | CDC." Centers for Disease Control and Prevention, October 25. https://www.cdc.gov/ncbddd/disabilityandhealth/materials/infographic-disabilities-ethnicity-race.html.

CDC. 2019. *"Infographic—Racial and Ethnic Disparities in Cardiovascular Disease."* Health, United States Spotlight, May.

CDC. 2019. *"Know Your Risk for Cardiovascular disease."* Centers for Disease Control and Prevention, December 9. https://www.cdc.gov/heartdisease/risk_factors.htm.

CDC. 2020. "Sleep and Sleep Disorders." *Centers for Disease Control and Prevention,* April 15. https://www.cdc.gov/sleep/index.html.

CDC. 2022. *"Cardiovascular disease Facts."* Centers for Disease Control and Prevention, February 7. https://www.cdc.gov/heartdisease/facts.htm.

CDC. 2022. *"COVID-19 and Your Health."* Centers for Disease Control and Prevention, February 25. https://www.cdc.gov/coronavirus/2019-ncov/need-extra-precautions/people-with-medical-conditions.html.

CDC. 2022. *"Family Health History of Cardiovascular disease | CDC."* Centers for Disease Control and Prevention, February 10. https://www.cdc.gov/genomics/disease/fh/history_heart_disease.htm.

CDC. 2022. "Hospitalization and Death by Race/Ethnicity." Centers for Disease Control and Prevention, March 10. https://www.cdc.gov/coronavirus/2019-ncov/covid-data/investigations-discovery/hospitalization-death-by-race-ethnicity.html.

CDCMMWR. 2019. "QuickStats: Age-Adjusted Death Rates from Diabetes Mellitus as Underlying or Contributing Cause Among Adults Aged ≥65 Years, by Race/Ethnicity—National Vital Statistics System, United States, 2004–2017." *Morbidity and Mortality Weekly Report 68.* https://doi.org/10.15585/mmwr.mm6824a6.

Center for Disease Control and Prevention. 2018. "Breast Cancer Rates Among Black Women and White Women." December 19, 2018. https://www.cdc.gov/cancer/breast/statistics/trends_invasive.htm.

Center for Disease Control and Prevention. 2020. "Hospitalization and Death by Race/Ethnicity." *Centers for Disease Control and Prevention.* February 11, 2020. https://www.cdc.gov/coronavirus/2019-ncov/covid-data/investigations-discovery/hospitalization-death-by-race-ethnicity.html.

Center for Disease Control and Prevention. 2022. "Covid Data Tracker." *Centers for Disease Control and Prevention.* May 31, 2022. https://covid.cdc.gov/covid-data-tracker/#demographics

Center for Disease Control and Prevention. 2022. "Health Equity Considerations & Racial & Ethnic Minority Groups." *Centers for Disease Control and Prevention.* January 25, 2022. https://www.cdc.gov/coronavirus/2019-ncov/community/health-equity/race-ethnicity.html.

Chadiha, Letha A., Portia Adams, David E. Biegel, Wendy Auslander, and Lorraine Gutierrez. 2004. "Empowering African American Women Informal Caregivers: A Literature Synthesis and Practice Strategies." *Social Work 49* (1): 97–108. https://doi.org/10.1093/sw/49.1.97.

Chappell, Bill. 2013. "California's Prison Sterilizations Reportedly Echo Eugenics Era." NPR, July 9, 2013, sec. America. https://www.npr.org/secti ons/thetwo-way/2013/07/09/200444613/californias-prison-sterilizations-reportedly-echoes-eugenics-era.

Chidi, Erica, and Erica P. Cahill. 2020. "Protecting Your Birth: A Guide for Black Mothers." *The New York Times*, October 22, 2020, sec. Parenting. https://www.nytimes.com/article/black-mothers-birth.html.

Chou, Roger, Gilbert J. Fanciullo, Perry G. Fine, Jeremy A. Adler, Jane C. Ballantyne, Pamela Davies, Marilee I. Donovan, et al. 2009. "Clinical Guidelines for the Use of Chronic Opioid Therapy in Chronic Noncancer Pain." *Journal of Pain 10*, no. 2 (February 1): 113–130.e22. https://doi.org/10.1016/j.jpain.2008.10.008.

Churchwell, Keith, Mitchell S. V. Elkind, Regina M. Benjamin, April P. Carson, Edward K. Chang, Willie Lawrence, Andrew Mills, et al. 2020. "Call to Action: Structural Racism as a Fundamental Driver of Health Disparities: A Presidential Advisory From the American Heart Association." *Circulation 142*, no. 24 (December 15): e454–68. https://doi.org/10.1161/CIR.00000 00000000936.

Clark, Luther T., and Umesh Lingegowda. 2005. "Acute Coronary Syndromes in Black Americans: Is Treatment Different? Should It Be?" *Current Cardiology Reports 7*, no. 4 (July): 249–54. https://doi.org/10.1007/s11 886-005-0045-z.

Clark, Rodney, Norman B. Anderson, Vernessa R. Clark, and David R. Williams. 1999. "Racism as a Stressor for African Americans: A Biopsychosocial Model." *American Psychologist* 54 (10): 805–16. https://doi. org/10.1037/0003-066X.54.10.805.

Colantonio, Lisandro D., Christopher M. Gamboa, Joshua S. Richman, Emily B. Levitan, Elsayed Z. Soliman, George Howard, and Monika M. Safford. 2017. "Black-White Differences in Incident Fatal, Nonfatal and Total Coronary Cardiovascular disease." *Circulation 136*, no. 2 (July 11): 152–66. https://doi.org/10.1161/CIRCULATIONAHA.116.025848.

Cole, W. Luke, and Sheila R. Foster. 2000. *From the Ground Up: Environmental Racism and the Rise of the Environmental Justice Movement*. New York: NYU Press.

Cooper, R., and R. David. 1986. "The Biological Concept of Race and Its Application to Public Health and Epidemiology." *Journal of Health Politics, Policy and Law 11* (1): 97–116. https://doi.org/10.1215/03616878-11-1-97.

Covey, Herbert C. 2008. *African-American Slave Medicine: Herbal and Non-Herbal Treatments*. Lanham: Lexington Books.

Crenshaw, Kimberle. 1989. "Demarginalizing the Intersection of Race and Sex: A Black Feminist Critique of Antidiscrimination Doctrine, Feminist Theory and Antiracist Politics." *University of Chicago Legal Forum1989* (1): 31.

Cucinotta, Domenico, and Maurizio Vanelli. 2020. "WHO Declares COVID-19 a Pandemic." *Acta Bio-Medica: Atenei Parmensis 91* (1): 157–60. https://doi.org/10.23750/abm.v91i1.9397.

Curry, Tommy J. 2017. *The Man-Not: Race, Class, Genre, and the Dilemmas of Black Manhood*. Philadelphia: Temple University Press.

Daniel, Diane. 2020. "A Stroke at 37 Meant Relearning Everything." www.heart.org, September 17. https://www.heart.org/en/news/2020/09/17/a-stroke-at-37-meant-relearning-everything.

Daniel, Diane. 2021. "The Night before a Big Presentation, Lawyer-Mother Has a Heart Attack." www.heart.org, February 2. https://www.heart.org/en/news/2021/02/02/the-night-before-a-big-presentation-lawyer-mother-has-a-heart-attack.

Davis, F. James. 1991. *Who Is Black? One Nation's Definition*. University Park: Pennsylvania State University Press.

Dean, Lorraine, and Roland J. Thorpe Jr. 2022. "What Structural Racism Is (or Is Not) and How to Measure It: Clarity for Public Health and Medical Researchers." *American Journal of Epidemiology* 191 (9): 1521–1526.

DeBerry, Jarvis. 2017. "When You Ignore Black People's Pain You Get a Mostly White Opioid Crisis | Opinion." *NOLA*, November 10. https://www.nola.com/opinions/article_886a3b60-20d5-5f4d-a680-4490ee084fe7.html.

Dionne, Evette. 2020. "What No One Tells Black Women About Cardiovascular disease." *ZORA* (blog), May 21. https://zora.medium.com/what-no-one-tells-black-women-about-heart-disease-af2c037eeae3.

Douglas, Erin. 2019. "Cancer Cluster Identified in Neighborhood near Union Pacific Rail Yard's Contamination." *Houston Chronicle, December 6*. https://www.houstonchronicle.com/business/article/Cancer-cluster-identified-in-Houston-neighborhood-14885972.php.

Dunkel Schetter, Christine, and Lynlee Tanner. 2012. "Anxiety, Depression and Stress in Pregnancy: Implications for Mothers, Children, Research, and Practice." *Current Opinion in Psychiatry 25* (2): 141–48. https://doi.org/10.1097/YCO.0b013e3283503680.

Dunlop, Dorothy D., Jing Song, John S. Lyons, Larry M. Manheim, and Rowland W. Chang. 2003. "Racial/Ethnic Differences in Rates of Depression among Preretirement Adults." *American Journal of Public Health 93*, no. 11 (November): 1945–52. https://doi.org/10.2105/ajph.93.11.1945.

Elflein, John. 2022. "Physical Inactivity Prevalence by Ethnicity U.S. 2020." Statista, February 17. https://www.statista.com/statistics/252063/us-sedentary-lifestyle-among-adults-by-ethnicity/.

Eligon, John, and Robert Gebeloff. 2016. "Affluent and Black, and Still Trapped by Segregation." *The New York Times*, August 20, 2016, sec. U.S. https://www.nytimes.com/2016/08/21/us/milwaukee-segregation-wealthy-black-families.html.

Equitable Housing Institute. 2019. "Exclusionary Housing Policies." *EHI—Equitable Housing Institute*. Accessed April 25. https://www.equitablehous ing.org/background/exclusionary-housing-practices/198-exclusionary-housing-practices.html.

Fingar, Kathryn R., Iris Mabry-Hernandez, Quyen Ngo-Metzger, Tracy Wolff, Claudia A. Steiner, and Anne Elixhauser. 2017. *"Delivery Hospitalizations Involving Preeclampsia and Eclampsia, 2005-2014 HCUP Statistical Brief #222."* May 2017. https://hcup-us.ahrq.gov/reports/statbriefs/sb222-Preeclampsia-Eclampsia-Delivery-Trends.jsp?utm_source=ahrq&utm _medium=en-1&utm_term=&utm_content=1&utm_campaign= ahrq_en4_25_2017.

Flack, J. M., S. A. Nasser, A. Goel, M. "Toni" Flowers, S. O'Connor, and E. Faucett. 2010. "Unmasking Racial/Ethnic Disparities in Cardiovascular Disease: Nutritional, Socioeconomic, Cultural, and Health-Care-Related Contributions." In *Cardiovascular Disease in Racial and Ethnic Minorities*, edited by Keith C. Ferdinand and Annemarie Armani, 51–79. Totowa, NJ: Humana Press. https://doi.org/10.1007/978-1-59745-410-0_3.

Forgiarini, Matteo, Marcello Gallucci, and Angelo Maravita. 2011. "Racism and the Empathy for Pain on Our Skin." *Frontiers in Psychology 2*. https://www.frontiersin.org/article/10.3389/fpsyg.2011.00108.

Freemon, Frank R. 1985. "The Health of the American Slave Examined by Means of Union Army Medical Statistics." *Journal of the National Medical Association 77*, no. 1 (January): 49–52.

Geronimus, Arline T. 1996. "Black/White Differences in the Relationship of Maternal Age to Birthweight: A Population-Based Test of the Weathering Hypothesis." *Social Science & Medicine* (1982) *42* (4): 589–97. https://doi.org/10.1016/0277-9536(95)00159-x.

Geronimus, Arline T., Margaret T. Hicken, Jay A. Pearson, Sarah J. Seashols, Kelly L. Brown, and Tracey Dawson Cruz. 2010. "Do US Black Women Experience Stress-Related Accelerated Biological Aging?" *Human Nature (Hawthorne, N.Y.) 21* (1): 19–38. https://doi.org/10.1007/s12 110-010-9078-0.

Gould, Elise, Janelle Jones, and Zane Mokhiber. 2018. "Black Workers Have Made No Progress in Closing Earnings Gaps with White Men since 2000." *Economic Policy Institute* (blog), September 12. https://www.epi.org/blog/black-workers-have-made-no-progress-in-closing-earnings-gaps-with-white-men-since-2000/.

Goyal, Monika K., Nathan Kuppermann, Sean D. Cleary, Stephen J. Teach, and James M. Chamberlain. 2015. "Racial Disparities in Clinical pain management of Children With Appendicitis in Emergency Departments." *JAMA Pediatrics 169*, no. 11 (November): 996–1002. https://doi.org/10.1001/jam apediatrics.2015.1915.

Graham, Garth N. 2016. "Why Your ZIP Code Matters More Than Your Genetic Code: Promoting Healthy Outcomes from Mother to Child." *Breastfeeding Medicine 11*, no. 8 (October): 396–97. https://doi.org/10.1089/bfm.2016.0113.

Graham, Garth. 2015. "Disparities in Cardiovascular Disease Risk in the United States." *Current Cardiology Reviews 11*, no. 3 (August): 238–45. https://doi.org/10.2174/1573403X11666141122220003.

Grandner, Michael A., Natasha J. Williams, Kristen L. Knutson, Dorothy Roberts, and Girardin Jean-Louis. 2016. "Sleep Disparity, Race/Ethnicity, and Socioeconomic Position." *Sleep Medicine 18* (February): 7–18. https://doi.org/10.1016/j.sleep.2015.01.020.

Gravlee, Clarence. 2021. "How Whiteness Works: JAMA and the Refusals of White Supremacy." *Somatosphere* (blog), March 27. http://somatosphere.net/2021/how-whiteness-works.html/.

Green, Carmen R., Karen O. Anderson, Tamara A. Baker, Lisa C. Campbell, Sheila Decker, Roger B. Fillingim, Donna A. Kalauokalani, et al. 2003. "The Unequal Burden of Pain: Confronting Racial and Ethnic Disparities in Pain." *Pain Medicine (Malden, Mass.) 4*, no. 3 (September): 277–94. https://doi.org/10.1046/j.1526-4637.2003.03034.x.

Green, Carmen Reneé, Tamara A. Baker, Edna M. Smith, and Yuka Sato. 2003. "The Effect of Race in Older Adults Presenting for Chronic Clinical pain management: A Comparative Study of Black and White Americans." *Journal of Pain 4*, no. 2 (March): 82–90. https://doi.org/10.1054/jpai.2003.8.

Grineski, Sara E., and Timothy W. Collins. 2018. "Geographic and Social Disparities in Exposure to Air Neurotoxicants at U.S. Public Schools." *Environmental Research 161* (February): 580–87. https://doi.org/10.1016/j.envres.2017.11.047.

Gruver, Jackson. 2019. "Racial Wage Gap for Men." Payscale—Salary Comparison, Salary Survey, Search Wages, May 7. https://www.payscale.com/research-and-insights/racial-wage-gap-for-men/.

Guerra, Maria. 2013. "Fact Sheet: The State of African American Women in the United States." Center for American Progress (blog). November 7, 2013. https://www.americanprogress.org/article/fact-sheet-the-state-of-african-american-women-in-the-united-states/.

Hagiwara, Nao, Richard B. Slatcher, Susan Eggly, and Louis A. Penner. 2017. "Physician Racial Bias and Word Use during Racially Discordant Medical Interactions." *Health Communication 32*, no. 4 (April): 401–8. https://doi.org/10.1080/10410236.2016.1138389.

Hale, Lauren, and Benjamin Hale. 2010. "Treat the Source Not the Symptoms: Why Thinking about Sleep Informs the Social Determinants of Health." *Health Education Research 25*, no. 3 (June): 395–400. https://doi.org/10.1093/her/cyq027.

Hale, Lauren, Terrence D. Hill, Elliot Friedman, F. Javier Nieto, Loren W. Galvao, Corinne D. Engelman, Kristen M. C. Malecki, and Paul E. Peppard. 2013. "Perceived Neighborhood Quality, Sleep Quality, and Health Status: Evidence from the Survey of the Health of Wisconsin." *Social Science & Medicine (1982) 79* (February): 16–22. https://doi.org/10.1016/j.socsci med.2012.07.021.

Hammond, Wizdom Powell, Derrick Matthews, and Giselle Corbie-Smith. 2010. "Psychosocial Factors Associated With Routine Health Examination Scheduling and Receipt Among African American Men." *Journal of the National Medical Association 102*, no. 4 (April 1): 276–89. https://doi.org/10.1016/S0027-9684(15)30600-3.

Hardeman, Rachel R., Katy A. Murphy, J'Mag Karbeah, and Katy Backes Kozhimannil. 2018. "Naming Institutionalized Racism in the Public Health Literature: A Systematic Literature Review." *Public Health Reports 133*, no. 3 (May 1): 240–49. https://doi.org/10.1177/0033354918760574.

Harrell, Jules P., Sadiki Hall, and James Taliaferro. 2003. "Physiological Responses to Racism and Discrimination: An Assessment of the Evidence." *American Journal of Public Health 93* (2): 243–48. https://doi.org/10.2105/AJPH.93.2.243.

Harris-Perry, Melissa Victoria. 2011. *Sister Citizen: Shame, Stereotypes, and Black Women in America*; [for Colored Girls Who've Considered Politics When Being Strong Isn't Enough]. New Haven, CT: Yale University Press.

Hausmann, Leslie R. M., Shasha Gao, Edward S. Lee, and Kent C. Kwoh. 2013. "Racial Disparities in the Monitoring of Patients on Chronic Opioid Therapy." *Pain 154* (1): 46–52. https://doi.org/10.1016/j.pain.2012.07.034.

Hayford, Vanessa. 2018. "The Humble History of Soul Food." *Black Foodie.* January 22. https://www.blackfoodie.co/the-humble-history-of-soul-food/.

HBCU Editors. 2014. "Black Women Are Ranked the Most Educated Group by Race & Gender." HBCU Buzz (blog). March 4, 2014. https://hbcubuzz.com/2014/03/black-women-are-ranked-the-most-educated-group-by-race-gender/.

Heckler, Margaret M. 1985. *Report of the Secretary's Task Force Report on Black and Minority Health Volume I: Executive Summary.* U.S. Department of Health and Human Services.

Hicken, Margaret T., Hedwig Lee, Jennifer Ailshire, Sarah A. Burgard, and David R. Williams. 2013. "'Every Shut Eye, Ain't Sleep': The Role of Racism-Related Vigilance in Racial/Ethnic Disparities in Sleep Difficulty." *Race and Social Problems 5* (2): 100–12. https://doi.org/10.1007/s12552-013-9095-9.

Hines, Anika L., and Roland J. Thorpe. 2019. "Abstract 002: Racial Disparities in Hypertension Among Young, Black and White Women, 1999-2014 National Health and Nutrition Examination Surveys." *Hypertension 74*, no. Suppl_1 (September): A002–A002. https://doi.org/10.1161/hyp.74.suppl_1.002.

Ho, Karen. 2021. "The US Economic Recovery Is Skipping Black and Hispanic Women." *Quartz.* January 11, 2021. https://qz.com/1955437/black-and-hispanic-women-continued-to-lose-jobs-in-december/.

Hoberman, John. 2012. *Black and Blue: The Origins and Consequences of Medical Racism.* Los Angeles: University of California Press.

Hoffman, Kelly M., Sophie Trawalter, Jordan R. Axt, and M. Norman Oliver. 2016. "Racial Bias in Pain Assessment and Treatment Recommendations, and False Beliefs about Biological Differences between Blacks and Whites." *Proceedings of the National Academy of Sciences of the United States of America 113* (16): 4296–4301. https://doi.org/10.1073/pnas.1516047113.

Hoffman, Kelly M., Sophie Trawalter, Jordan R. Axt, and M. Norman Oliver. 2016. "Racial Bias in Pain Assessment and Treatment Recommendations, and False Beliefs about Biological Differences between Blacks and Whites." *Proceedings of the National Academy of Sciences of the United States of America 113,* no. 16 (April 19): 4296–4301. https://doi.org/10.1073/pnas.1516047113.

Holland, Brynn. 2018. "The 'Father of Modern Gynecology' Performed Shocking Experiments on Enslaved Women." *HISTORY.* 2018. https://www.history.com/news/the-father-of-modern-gynecology-performed-shocking-experiments-on-slaves.

Holloway, Karla F. C. 2011. *Private Bodies, Public Texts: Race, Gender, and a Cultural Bioethics.* Durham, NC: Duke University Press

Holzer, Harry J. 2021. "Why Are Employment Rates so Low among Black Men?" *Brookings* (blog), March 1. https://www.brookings.edu/research/why-are-employment-rates-so-low-among-black-men/.

Howell, Elizabeth A. 2018. "Reducing Disparities in Severe Maternal Morbidity and Mortality." *Clinical Obstetrics and Gynecology 61* (2): 387–99. https://doi.org/10.1097/GRF.0000000000000349.

Howell, Elizabeth A., Jennifer Zeitlin, Paul L. Hebert, Amy Balbierz, and Natalia Egorova. 2014. "Association between Hospital-Level Obstetric Quality Indicators and Maternal and Neonatal Morbidity." *JAMA 312* (15): 1531–41. https://doi.org/10.1001/jama.2014.13381.

Howell, Elizabeth A., Natalia Egorova, Amy Balbierz, Jennifer Zeitlin, and Paul L. Hebert. 2016. "Black-White Differences in Severe Maternal Morbidity and Site of Care." *American Journal of Obstetrics and Gynecology 214* (1): 122.e1–122.e7. https://doi.org/10.1016/j.ajog.2015.08.019.

IMDb. "John Singleton." Accessed March 19, 2022. http://www.imdb.com/name/nm0005436/awards.

Institute of Medicine (US) Committee on Advancing Pain Research, Care, and Education. 2011. *Relieving Pain in America: A Blueprint for Transforming Prevention, Care, Education, and Research. The National Academies Collection: Reports Funded by National Institutes of Health.* Washington

(DC): National Academies Press (US). http://www.ncbi.nlm.nih.gov/books/NBK91497/.

Institute of Medicine (US) Committee on Understanding and Eliminating Racial and Ethnic Disparities in Health Care. 2003. *Unequal Treatment: Confronting Racial and Ethnic Disparities in Health Care.* Edited by Brian D. Smedley, Adrienne Y. Stith, and Alan R. Nelson. Washington, DC: National Academies Press (US). http://www.ncbi.nlm.nih.gov/books/NBK220358/.

Jackson, Chandra L., Susan Redline, and Karen M. Emmons. 2015. "Sleep as a Potential Fundamental Contributor to Disparities in Cardiovascular Health." *Annual Review of Public Health 36* (March 18): 417–40. https://doi.org/10.1146/annurev-publhealth-031914-122838.

Jackson, Chandra L., Susan Redline, Ichiro Kawachi, Michelle A. Williams, and Frank B. Hu. 2013. "Racial Disparities in Short Sleep Duration by Occupation and Industry." *American Journal of Epidemiology 178*, no. 9 (November 1): 1442–51. https://doi.org/10.1093/aje/kwt159.

JAMA Network. *Structural Racism in Medicine and Health Care,* 2021. https://www.youtube.com/watch?v=SyzZvlvoAys.

Jama, Riya. 2018. "Doctors Refused to Diagnose My Chronic Illness Because This World Ignores Black Women's Pain." *The Black Youth Project* (blog), October 16. http://blackyouthproject.com/doctors-refused-to-diagnose-my-chronic-illness-because-this-world-ignores-black-womens-pain/.

JAMA. 2021. "Statement from Howard Bauchner, MD, Editor in Chief JAMA and The JAMA Network Https://T.Co/A1AJNnMWB4." Tweet. *@JAMA_current* (blog), March 4. https://twitter.com/JAMA_current/status/1367546743789862912.

Jaschik, Scott. 2017. "Anger Over Stereotypes in Textbook." Inside Higher Ed, October 23. https://www.insidehighered.com/news/2017/10/23/nursing-textbook-pulled-over-stereotypes.

Jolly, Stacey, Eric Vittinghoff, Arpita Chattopadhyay, and Kirsten Bibbins-Domingo. 2010. "Higher Cardiovascular Disease Prevalence and Mortality among Younger Blacks Compared to Whites." *The American Journal of Medicine 123*, no. 9 (September 1): 811–18. https://doi.org/10.1016/j.amjmed.2010.04.020.

Kahn, Jonathan. 2012. *Race in a Bottle: The Story of BiDil and Racialized Medicine in a Post-Genomic Age.* Columbia University Press.

Kaine, Tim. 2020. "S.4269—116th Congress (2019-2020): Mothers and Newborns Success Act." Legislation. 2019/2020. July 22, 2020. https://www.congress.gov/bill/116th-congress/senate-bill/4269.

Kaiser Family Foundation. 2021. "Number of Diabetes Deaths per 100,000 Population by Race/Ethnicity." *KFF* (blog), March 16. https://www.kff.org/other/state-indicator/diabetes-death-rate-by-raceethnicity/.

Kaiser Family Foundation. 2021. "State Health Facts: Number of Deaths per 100,000 Population by Race/Ethnicity." *KFF* (blog), March 16. https://www.kff.org/other/state-indicator/death-rate-by-raceethnicity/.

Kaplan, Jonathan. 2019. "Self-Care as Self Blame Redux: Stress as Personal and Political." *Kennedy Institute of Ethics Journal 29*, no. 2 (June): 97–123.

Kawai, Kosuke, Alison Tse Kawai, Peter Wollan, and Barbara P. Yawn. 2017. "Adverse Impacts of Chronic Pain on Health-Related Quality of Life, Work Productivity, Depression and Anxiety in a Community-Based Study." *Family Practice 34*, no. 6 (November 16): 656–61. https://doi.org/10.1093/fampra/cmx034.

Keel, Terence. 2018. *Divine Variations: How Christian Thought Became Racial Science.* Stanford: Stanford University Press.

Kelley, P., and P. Clifford. 1997. "Coping with Chronic Pain: Assessing Narrative Approaches." *Social Work 42*, no. 3 (May): 266–77. https://doi.org/10.1093/sw/42.3.266.

Kenny, Stephen C. 2016. "Medical Racism's Poison Pen: The Toxic World of Dr. Henry Ramsay (1821–1856)." *The Southern Quarterly 54*, nos. 3–4: 70–96.

Khanna, Nikki. 2016. "'If You're Half Black, You're Just Black': Reflected Appraisals and the Persistence of the One-Drop Rule." *The Sociological Quarterly 51* (1): 96–121. https://doi.org/10.1111/j.1533-8525.2009.01162.x.

Kingsbury, John H., Orfeu M. Buxton, and Karen M. Emmons. 2013. "Sleep and Its Relationship to Racial and Ethnic Disparities in Cardiovascular Disease." *Current Cardiovascular Risk Reports 7*, no. 5 (October): 10.1007/s12170-013-0330-0. https://doi.org/10.1007/s12170-013-0330-0.

Kingsbury, John H., Orfeu M. Buxton, and Karen M. Emmons. 2013. "Sleep and Its Relationship to Racial and Ethnic Disparities in Cardiovascular Disease." *Current Cardiovascular Risk Reports 7*, no. 5 (October): 10.1007/s12170-013-0330-0. https://doi.org/10.1007/s12170-013-0330-0.

Kirsch, B., H. Berdine, D. Zablotsky, G. Wenzel, and C. Meyer. 2000. "Implementation of a Clinical pain management Strategy: Identifying Pain as the Fifth Vital Sign," no. 5: 49–59.

Krefetz, Sharon Perlman. 1979. "Low- and Moderate-Income Housing in the Suburbs: The Massachusetts 'Anti-Snob Zoning' Law Experience." *Policy Studies Journal 8*, no. 2: 288–99. https://doi.org/10.1111/j.1541-0072.1979.tb01580.x.

Krieger, N. 1987. "Shades of Difference: Theoretical Underpinnings of the Medical Controversy on Black/White Differences in the United States, 1830–1870." *International Journal of Health Services: Planning, Administration, Evaluation 17* (2): 259–78. https://doi.org/10.2190/DBY6-VDQ8-HME8-ME3R.

Krieger, N. 2001. "The Ostrich, the Albatross, and Public Health: An Ecosocial Perspective—or Why an Explicit Focus on Health Consequences of

Discrimination and Deprivation Is Vital for Good Science and Public Health Practice." *Public Health Reports 116* (5): 419–23.

Krieger, Nancy, Rhea W Boyd, Fernando De Maio, and Aletha Maybank. 2021. "Medicine's Privileged Gatekeepers: Producing Harmful Ignorance About Racism and Health | Health Affairs Forefront," April 20. https://www.health affairs.org/do/10.1377/forefront.20210415.305480/full/.

Kristof, Nicholas. 2020. "What If There Were No George Floyd Video?" *The New York Times*, June 6, sec. Opinion. https://www.nytimes.com/2020/06/06/opinion/sunday/george-floyd-structural-racism.html.

Kuta, Sarah. 2022. "Subjected to Painful Experiments and Forgotten, Enslaved 'Mothers of Gynecology' Are Honored With New Monument." *Smithsonian*. https://www.smithsonianmag.com/smart-news/mothers-of-gynecology-monument-honors-enslaved-women-180980064/

Lake, Jaboa. 2020. "The Pandemic Has Exacerbated Housing Instability for Renters of Color." Center for American Progress (blog). October 30, 2020. https://www.americanprogress.org/article/pandemic-exacerbated-housing-instability-renters-color/.

Laposky, Aaron D., Eve Van Cauter, and Ana V. Diez-Roux. 2016. "Reducing Health Disparities: The Role of Sleep Deficiency and Sleep Disorders." *Sleep Medicine 18* (February): 3–6. https://doi.org/10.1016/j.sleep.2015.01.007.

Lartey, Jamiles, and Oliver Laughland. "'Almost Every Household Has Someone That Has Died from Cancer.'" *The Guardian*, 20119-05-06. http://www.theguardian.com/us-news/ng-interactive/2019/may/06/cancertown-louisana-reserve-special-report.

Lauderdale, Diane S., Kristen L. Knutson, Lijing L. Yan, Paul J. Rathouz, Stephen B. Hulley, Steve Sidney, and Kiang Liu. 2006. "Objectively Measured Sleep Characteristics among Early-Middle-Aged Adults: The CARDIA Study." *American Journal of Epidemiology 164*, no. 1 (July 1): 5–16. https://doi.org/10.1093/aje/kwj199.

Leifheit-Limson, Erica C., John A. Spertus, Kimberly J. Reid, Sara B. Jones, Viola Vaccarino, Harlan M. Krumholz, and Judith H. Lichtman. 2013. "Prevalence of Traditional Cardiac Risk Factors and Secondary Prevention among Patients Hospitalized for Acute Myocardial Infarction (AMI): Variation by Age, Sex, and Race." *Journal of Women's Health (2002) 22*, no. 8 (August): 659–66. https://doi.org/10.1089/jwh.2012.3962.

Leonhardt, David. 2015. "Middle-Class Black Families, in Low-Income Neighborhoods." *The New York Times*, June 24, sec. The Upshot. https://www.nytimes.com/2015/06/25/upshot/middle-class-black-families-in-low-income-neighborhoods.html.

Li, Jing, and Judith Scott-Clayton. 2016. "Black-White Disparity in Student Loan Debt More than Triples after Graduation." Brookings (blog). October 20, 2016. https://www.brookings.edu/research/black-white-disparity-in-student-loan-debt-more-than-triples-after-graduation/.

Livingston, Ed. 2021. "Part 3: Interview with Dr. Mitch Katz and Host Ed Livingston (Transcript)," May 5. https://static1.squarespace.com/static/5d7d985bfc6bb40f1dfae872/t/6061d1425689961a044a3ac0/1617023298545/Transcript+-+Structural+Racism+for+Doctors.pdf.

Lockhart, P. R. 2018. "What Serena Williams's Scary Childbirth Story Says about Medical Treatment of Black Women." *Vox.* January 11, 2018. https://www.vox.com/identities/2018/1/11/16879984/serena-williams-childbirth-scare-black-women.

Long, Margaret Geneva. 2012. *Doctoring Freedom: The Politics of African American Medical Care in Slavery and Emancipation. John Hope Franklin Series in African American History and Culture.* Chapel Hill: University of North Carolina Press.

Lu, Michael C. 2018. "Reducing Maternal Mortality in the United States." *JAMA 320* (12): 1237–38. https://doi.org/10.1001/jama.2018.11652.

Lujan, Heidi L., and Stephen E. DiCarlo. 2018. "The 'African Gene' Theory: It Is Time to Stop Teaching and Promoting the Slavery Hypertension Hypothesis." *Advances in Physiology Education 42,* no. 3 (September): 412–16. https://doi.org/10.1152/advan.00070.2018.

Lurie, Nicole, Allen Fremont, Arvind K. Jain, Stephanie L. Taylor, Rebecca McLaughlin, Eric Peterson, B. Waine Kong, and T. Bruce Ferguson. 2005. "Racial and Ethnic Disparities in Care: The Perspectives of Cardiologists." *Circulation 111,* no. 10 (March 15): 1264–69. https://doi.org/10.1161/01.CIR.0000157738.12783.71.

Magnan, Sanne. 2017. "Social Determinants of Health 101 for Health Care: Five Plus Five." *NAM Perspectives,* October 9. https://doi.org/10.31478/201710c.

Mainous, Arch G., Rebecca J. Tanner, Ara Jo, Ki Park, and V. Madsen Beau De Rochars. 2018. "Trends in Cardiovascular Disease Risk in the U.S., 1999–2014." *American Journal of Preventive Medicine 55,* no. 3 (September 1): 384–88. https://doi.org/10.1016/j.amepre.2018.04.025.

Marta, Suzanne. 2021. "Doctor Asked, 'Did You Know You Had a Heart Attack?'" www.heart.org, April 23. https://www.heart.org/en/news/2021/04/23/doctor-asked-did-you-know-you-had-a-heart-attack.

Martin, Nina, and Julia Belluz. 2019. "Lost Mothers." *ProPublica.* May 25, 2019. https://www.propublica.org/series/lost-mothers?token=aGn0cAzF1vcRrdeL0ElVR2hgvgtEPpJo.

Martin, Nina, and Renee Montagne. 2017. "Nothing Protects Black Women From Dying in Pregnancy and Childbirth." *ProPublica. 2017.* https://www.propublica.org/article/nothing-protects-black-women-from-dying-in-pregnancy-and-childbirth?token=Q9-9suvCib74rpcNfQRtz25BIr6KF0ah.

Martinez, Emmanuel and Lauren Kirchner. 2021. "The Secret Bias Hidden in Mortgage-Approval Algorithms." *The Markup,* August 25, https://themarkup.org/denied/2021/08/25/the-secret-bias-hidden-in-mortgage-approval-algorithms.

McCargo, Alanna. 2019. "A Five-Point Strategy for Reducing the Black Homeownership Gap." *Urban Institute*. February 14. https://www.urban. org/urban-wire/five-point-strategy-reducing-black-homeownership-gap.

McFarling, Usha Lee. 2021. "Troubling Podcast Puts JAMA, the 'voice of Medicine,' under Fire for Its Mishandling of Race." *STAT* (blog), April 6. https://www.statnews.com/2021/04/06/podcast-puts-jama-under-fire-for-mishandling-of-race/.

McKinsey & Company. 2021. "*Women in the Workplace 2021.*" https://www. mckinsey.com/featured-insights/diversity-and-inclusion/women-in-the-workplace.

MedlinePlus Genetics. 2020. "Sickle Cell Disease." *National Library of Medicine*. August 18, 2020. https://medlineplus.gov/genetics/condition/sic kle-cell-disease/.

Meghani, Salimah H., Eeeseung Byun, and Rollin M. Gallagher. 2012. "Time to Take Stock: A Meta-Analysis and Systematic Review of Analgesic Treatment Disparities for Pain in the United States." *Pain Medicine (Malden, Mass.)* 13, no. 2 (February): 150–74. https://doi.org/10.1111/ j.1526-4637.2011.01310.x.

Mensah, George A. 2018. "Cardiovascular Diseases in African Americans: Fostering Community Partnerships to Stem the Tide." *American Journal of Kidney Diseases: The Official Journal of the National Kidney Foundation 72*, no. 5 Suppl 1 (November): S37–42. https://doi.org/ 10.1053/j.ajkd.2018.06.026.

Mezick, Elizabeth J., Karen A. Matthews, Martica Hall, Patrick J. Strollo, Daniel J. Buysse, Thomas W. Kamarck, Jane F. Owens, and Steven E. Reis. 2008. "Influence of Race and Socioeconomic Status on Sleep: Pittsburgh Sleep SCORE Project." *Psychosomatic Medicine 70*, no. 4 (May): 410–16. https:// doi.org/10.1097/PSY.0b013e31816fdf21.

Mills, Charles W. 2005. "'Ideal Theory' as Ideology." *Hypatia 20*, no. 3: 165–84. https://doi.org/10.1353/hyp.2005.0107.

Moffett-Bateau, Alexandra. 2014. "Chronic Pain, and the Denial of Care for Black Women." Rewire News Group, March 4. https://rewire.news/article/ 2014/03/04/chronic-pain-denial-care-black-women/.

Morden, Nancy E., Deanna Chyn, Andrew Wood, and Ellen Meara. 2021. "Racial Inequality in Prescription Opioid Receipt—Role of Individual Health Systems." *New England Journal of Medicine 385*, no. 4 (July 22): 342– 51. https://doi.org/10.1056/NEJMsa2034159.

Mossey, Jana M. 2011. "Defining Racial and Ethnic Disparities in Pain Management." *Clinical Orthopaedics and Related Research 469* (7): 1859–70. https://doi.org/10.1007/s11999-011-1770-9.

Mularski, Richard A., Foy White-Chu, Devorah Overbay, Lois Miller, Steven M. Asch, and Linda Ganzini. 2006. "Measuring Pain as the 5th Vital Sign Does Not Improve Quality of Clinical pain management." *Journal of*

General Internal Medicine 21, no. 6 (June): 607–12. https://doi.org/10.1111/j.1525-1497.2006.00415.x.

Mumba, Pie. "Serena Williams' Birthing Scare Highlights Poor Black Maternal Health." *Longevity.* https://longevitylive.com/wellness/serena-williams-birthing-scare-highlights-poor-black-maternal-health/.

Naftulin, Julia. 2020. *"Inside the Hidden Campaign to Forcibly Sterilize Thousands of Inmates in California Women's Prisons." Insider.* https://www.insider.com/inside-forced-sterilizations-california-womens-prisons-documentary-2020-11.

National Human Genome Research Institute. 2018. "Genetics vs. Genomics Fact Sheet." September 7, 2018. https://www.genome.gov/about-genomics/fact-sheets/Genetics-vs-Genomics.

NEJM Group. 2021. "Racial Disparities in Clinical Medicine: Conversations, Perspectives, and Research on Advancing Medical Equity." Massachusetts Medical Society. https://store.nejm.org/media/assets/nejm/register/pdf/NEJM_Group_Racial_Disparities_in_Clinical_Medicine.pdf.

Niles, George M. 1913. "A Therapeutic Comparison, Medicinal and Otherwise, as Between the Caucasian and Afro-American." *Southern Medical Journal*, no. 6: 128.

North, Anna. 2020. "America Is Failing Black Moms during the Pandemic." *Vox.* August 10, 2020. https://www.vox.com/2020/8/10/21336312/covid-19-pregnancy-birth-black-maternal-mortality.

Nunes, Joao, Girardin Jean-Louis, Ferdinand Zizi, Georges J. Casimir, Hans von Gizycki, Clinton D. Brown, and Samy I. McFarlane. 2008. "Sleep Duration among Black and White Americans: Results of the National Health Interview Survey." *Journal of the National Medical Association 100*, no. 3 (March): 317–22. https://doi.org/10.1016/s0027-9684(15)31244-x.

Nunez, Kirsten, and Karen Lamoreux. 2020. "Why Do We Sleep?" *Healthline*, July 20. https://www.healthline.com/health/why-do-we-sleep.

Office of Disease Prevention and Health Promotion. 2014. "Social Determinants of Health." *HealthyPeople.Gov.* 2014. https://www.healthypeople.gov/2020/topics-objectives/topic/social-determinants-of-health.

Olafiranye, Oladipupo, Olakunle Akinboboye, Judith Mitchell, Gbenga Ogedegbe, and Girardin Jean-Louis. 2013. "Obstructive Sleep Apnea and Cardiovascular Disease in Blacks: A Call to Action from Association of Black Cardiologists." *American Heart Journal 165*, no. 4 (April): 468–76. https://doi.org/10.1016/j.ahj.2012.12.018.

Oluo, Ijeoma. 2018. *So You Want to Talk about* Race. First edition. New York: Seal Press.

Omeish, Yousof, and Samantha Kiernan. 2020. "Targeting Bias to Improve Maternal Care and Outcomes for Black Women in the USA." *EClinicalMedicine* 27 (October). https://doi.org/10.1016/j.eclinm.2020.100568.

Orminski, Emily. 2021. "Your Zip Code Is More Important than Your Genetic Code » NCRC," June 30. https://www.ncrc.org/your-zip-code-is-more-important-than-your-genetic-code/.

Owens, Deirdre Cooper, and Sharla M. Fett. 2019. "Black Maternal and Infant Health: Historical Legacies of Slavery." *American Journal of Public Health* 109 (10): 1342–45. https://doi.org/10.2105/AJPH.2019.305243.

Paradies, Yin, Jehonathan Ben, Nida Denson, Amanuel Elias, Naomi Priest, Alex Pieterse, Arpana Gupta, Margaret Kelaher, and Gilbert Gee. 2015. "Racism as a Determinant of Health: A Systematic Review and Meta-Analysis." *PLoS ONE 10*, no. 9 (September 23): e0138511. https://doi.org/10.1371/journal.pone.0138511.

Patel, Nirav P., Michael A. Grandner, Dawei Xie, Charles C. Branas, and Nalaka Gooneratne. 2010. " 'Sleep Disparity' in the Population: Poor Sleep Quality Is Strongly Associated with Poverty and Ethnicity." *BMC Public Health 10*, no. 1 (August 11): 475. https://doi.org/10.1186/1471-2458-10-475.

Payscale. n.d. "The State of the Gender Pay Gap in 2021." Payscale—Salary Comparison, Salary Survey, Search Wages. https://www.payscale.com/research-and-insights/gender-pay-gap/.

Pierce, Jacob B, Kiarri N. Kershaw, Catarina I. Kiefe, et al. 2020. "Association of Childhood Psychosocial Environment With a 30-Year Cardiovascular Disease Incidence and Mortality in Middle Age." *Journal of the American Heart Association 9* (9): e015326.

Pollack, Craig Evan, Sekai Chideya, Catherine Cubbin, Brie Williams, Mercedes Dekker, and Paula Braveman. 2007. "Should Health Studies Measure Wealth? A Systematic Review." *American Journal of Preventive Medicine 33* (3): 250–64. https://doi.org/10.1016/j.amepre.2007.04.033.

Presser, Lizzie. 2020. "The Black American Amputation Epidemic." ProPublica, May 19. https://features.propublica.org/diabetes-amputations/black-american-amputation-epidemic/.

Public Health Agency of Canada. 2020. "Social Determinants of Health and Health Inequalities." *Government of Canada*. October 7, 2020. https://www.canada.ca/en/public-health/services/health-promotion/population-health/what-determines-health.html.

Quenqua, Douglas. 2012. "How Well You Sleep May Hinge on Race." *The New York Times*, August 20, sec. Health. https://www.nytimes.com/2012/08/21/health/how-well-you-sleep-may-hinge-on-race.html.

Quinn, Kay. 2018. "Moms of Color Say They're Terrified of Dying in Childbirth and No One Is Listening." Ksdk.Com. October 24, 2018. https://www.ksdk.com/article/news/investigations/mothers-matter/moms-of-color-say-theyre-terrified-of-dying-in-childbirth-and-no-one-is-listening/63-607056009.

Ray, Keisha. 2016. "Blog—Inefficient Clinical pain management for Black Patients Shows That There Is a Fine Line between 'Inhumane' and

'Superhuman.'" *Bioethics Today*, May 4. https://bioethicstoday.org/blog/inefficient-pain-management-for-black-patients-shows-that-there-is-a-fine-line-between-inhumane-and-superhuman/.

Ray, Keisha. 2017. "Intersectionality and the Dangers of White Empathy When Treating Black Patients." *Bioethics Today*. 2017. https://bioethicstoday.org/blog/intersectionality-and-the-dangers-of-white-empathy-when-treating-black-patients/.

Ray, Keisha. 2018. "Blog—Black Women Are Dying in Disproportionate Numbers During and After Giving Birth and Not Even Celebrity Serena Williams Is Safe." *Bioethics Today*. January 16, 2018. https://bioethicstoday.org/blog/black-women-are-dying-in-disproportionate-numbers-during-and-after-giving-birth-and-not-even-celebrity-serena-williams-is-safe/.

Ray, Keisha. 2021. "Black and Sleepless in a Nonideal World." In *Applying Nonideal Theory to Bioethics: Living and Dying in a Nonideal World*, edited by Elizabeth Victor and Laura K. Guidry-Grimes, 235–54. Springer.

Ray, Keisha. 2021. "In the Name of Racial Justice: Why Bioethics Should Care About Environmental Toxins." *Hastings Center Report 51*, no. 3: 23–26. https://doi.org/10.1002/hast.1251.

Reaves, Stephanie. 2021. "Mental Health Association in Delaware." *Minority Mental Health Month* (blog), July 5. https://www.mhainde.org/minority-mental-health-month/.

Reeves, Richard, Edward Rodrigue, and Elizabeth Kneebone. 2016. "Five Evils: Multidimensional Poverty and Race in America." *The Brookings Institution*, April, https://www.brookings.edu/wp-content/uploads/2016/06/reeveskneebonerodrigue_multidimensionalpoverty_fullpaper.pdf.

Resnick, Brian. 2015. "The Racial Inequality of Sleep." *The Atlantic*, October 27. https://www.theatlantic.com/health/archive/2015/10/the-sleep-gap-and-racial-inequality/412405/.

Riddell, Corinne A., Kathryn T. Morrison, Jay S. Kaufman, and Sam Harper. 2018. "Trends in the Contribution of Major Causes of Death to the Black-White Life Expectancy Gap by US State." *Health & Place 52* (July): 85–100. https://doi.org/10.1016/j.healthplace.2018.04.003.

Roberts, Dorothy. 2011. *Fatal Invention: How Science, Politics, and Big Business Re-Create Race in the Twenty-First Century*. New York: New Press.

Roberts, Dorothy. 2017. *Killing the Black Body*. 2nd ed. New York: Vintage Books.

Roeder, Amy. 2019. "America Is Failing Its Black Mothers." *Harvard Public Health Magazine. 2019*. https://www.hsph.harvard.edu/magazine/magazine_article/america-is-failing-its-black-mothers/.

Romero, Lisa, Karen Pazol, Lee Warner, Shanna Cox, Charlan Kroelinger, Ghenet Besera, Anna Brittain, Taleria R. Fuller, Emilia Koumans, and Wanda Barfield. 2016. "Reduced Disparities in Birth Rates Among Teens Aged 15–19 Years—United States, 2006–2007 and 2013–2014." *Morbidity and Mortality Weekly Report 65* (16): 409–14.

Rose, Julie. 2012. "North Carolina Eugenics Victims Not Giving Up." NPR, August 17, 2012, sec. Law. https://www.npr.org/2012/08/17/158984357/ north-carolina-eugenics-victims-plan-next-steps.

Ross, Paula T., Monica L. Lypson, and Arno K. Kumagai. 2012. "Using Illness Narratives to Explore African American Perspectives of Racial Discrimination in Health Care." *Journal of Black Studies 43*, no. 5 (July 1): 520–44. https://doi.org/10.1177/0021934711436129.

Rothstein, Richard. 2017. *The Color of Law: A Forgotten History of How Our Government Segregated America. First edition.* New York; London: Liveright Publishing Corporation, a division of W. W. Norton & Company.

Rouse, Cecilia, Jared Bernstein, Helen Knudsen, and Jeffery Zhang. 2021. "Exclusionary Zoning: Its Effect on Racial Discrimination in the Housing Market." *The White House*, June 17. https://www.whitehouse.gov/cea/writ ten-materials/2021/06/17/exclusionary-zoning-its-effect-on-racial-dis crimination-in-the-housing-market/.

Rozanski, A., J. A. Blumenthal, and J. Kaplan. 1999. "Impact of Psychological Factors on the Pathogenesis of Cardiovascular Disease and Implications for Therapy." *Circulation 99*, no. 16 (April 27): 2192–2217. https://doi.org/ 10.1161/01.cir.99.16.2192.

Rucker-Whitaker, Cheryl, Joe Feinglass, and William H. Pearce. 2003. "Explaining Racial Variation in Lower Extremity Amputation: A 5-Year Retrospective Claims Data and Medical Record Review at an Urban Teaching Hospital." *Archives of Surgery 138*, no. 12 (December 1): 1347–51. https://doi.org/10.1001/archsurg.138.12.1347.

Ruiter, Megan E., Jamie Decoster, Lindsey Jacobs, and Kenneth L. Lichstein. 2011. "Normal Sleep in African-Americans and Caucasian-Americans: A Meta-Analysis." *Sleep Medicine 12*, no. 3 (March): 209–14. https://doi.org/ 10.1016/j.sleep.2010.12.010.

Ruiz-Grossman, Sarah. 2019. "California Takes New Steps To Stop Black Women From Dying In Childbirth." *HuffPost*. October 8, 2019. https:// www.huffpost.com/entry/california-bill-black-maternal-mortality_n_5 d9cd594e4b06ddfc50f6f0e.

Sabin, Janice, Brian A. Nosek, Anthony Greenwald, and Frederick P. Rivara. 2009. "Physicians' Implicit and Explicit Attitudes about Race by MD Race, Ethnicity, and Gender." *Journal of Health Care for the Poor and Underserved 20* (3): 896–913. https://doi.org/10.1353/hpu.0.0185.

Sacks, Tina K. 2019. *Invisible Visits: Black Middle Class Women in the American Healthcare System*. New York: Oxford University Press.

Saha, Somnath, and Mary Catherine Beach. 2020. "Impact of Physician Race on Patient Decision-Making and Ratings of Physicians: A Randomized Experiment Using Video Vignettes." *Journal of General Internal Medicine 35*, no. 4 (April 1): 1084–91. https://doi.org/10.1007/s11606-020-05646-z.

Schulman, Kevin A., Jesse A. Berlin, William Harless, Jon F. Kerner, Shyrl Sistrunk, Bernard J. Gersh, Ross Dubé, et al. 1999. "The Effect of Race and Sex on Physicians' Recommendations for Cardiac Catheterization." *New England Journal of Medicine 340*, no. 8 (February 25): 618–26. https://doi.org/10.1056/NEJM199902253400806.

Serafini, Kelly, Caitlin Coyer, Joedrecka Brown Speights, Dennis Donovan, Jessica Guh, Judy Washington, and Carla Ainsworth. 2020. "Racism as Experienced by Physicians of Color in the Health Care Setting." *Family Medicine 52*, no. 4: 282–87. https://doi.org/10.22454/FamMed.2020.384384.

Shah, Adil A., Cheryl K. Zogg, Syed Nabeel Zafar, Eric B. Schneider, Lisa A. Cooper, Alyssa B. Chapital, Susan M. Peterson, et al. 2015. "Analgesic Access for Acute Abdominal Pain in the Emergency Department Among Racial/Ethnic Minority Patients: A Nationwide Examination." *Medical Care 53*, no. 12 (December): 1000–1009. https://doi.org/10.1097/MLR.0000000000000444.

Shammas, Masood A. 2011. "Telomeres, Lifestyle, Cancer, and Aging." *Current Opinion in Clinical Nutrition and Metabolic Care* 14 (1): 28–34. https://doi.org/10.1097/MCO.0b013e32834121b1.

Singhal, Astha, Yu-Yu Tien, and Renee Y. Hsia. 2016. "Racial-Ethnic Disparities in Opioid Prescriptions at Emergency Department Visits for Conditions Commonly Associated with Prescription Drug Abuse." *PLOS ONE 11*, no. 8 (August 8): e0159224. https://doi.org/10.1371/journal.pone.0159224.

Skolarus, Lesli E., Anjail Sharrief, Hannah Gardener, Carolyn Jenkins, and Bernadette Boden-Albala. 2020. "Considerations in Addressing Social Determinants of Health to Reduce Racial/Ethnic Disparities in Stroke Outcomes in the United States." *Stroke 51*, no. 11 (November): 3433–39. https://doi.org/10.1161/STROKEAHA.120.030426.

Smedley, Audrey, and Brian D. Smedley. 2005. "Race as Biology Is Fiction, Racism as a Social Problem Is Real: Anthropological and Historical Perspectives on the Social Construction of Race." *The American Psychologist 60* (1): 16–26. https://doi.org/10.1037/0003-066X.60.1.16.

Staton, Lisa J., Mukta Panda, Ian Chen, Inginia Genao, James Kurz, Mark Pasanen, Alex J. Mechaber, et al. 2007. "When Race Matters: Disagreement in Pain Perception between Patients and Their Physicians in Primary Care." *Journal of the National Medical Association 99*, no. 5 (May): 532–38.

Sternthal, Michelle J., Natalie Slopen, and David R. Williams. 2011. "Racial Disparities in Health: How Much Does Stress Really Matter?." *Du Bois Review: Social Science Research on Race 8* (1): 95–113. https://doi.org/10.1017/S1742058X11000087.

Strumpf, Erin C. 2011. "Racial/Ethnic Disparities in Primary Care: The Role of Physician-Patient Concordance." *Medical Care 49*, no. 5 (May): 496–503. https://doi.org/10.1097/MLR.0b013e31820fbee4.

Sullivan, Shannon. 2015. *The Physiology of Sexist and Racist Oppression. Studies in Feminist Philosophy.* Oxford; New York: Oxford University Press.

Sun, Michael, Tomasz Oliwa, Monica E. Peek, and Elizabeth L. Tung. 2022. "Negative Patient Descriptors: Documenting Racial Bias In The Electronic Health Record: Study Examines Racial Bias in the Patient Descriptors Used in the Electronic Health Record." *Health Affairs 41* (2): 203–11. https://doi.org/10.1377/hlthaff.2021.01423.

Suni, Eric. 2017. "Sleep Disorders and Race: What's the Connection?" *Sleep Foundation,* November 4. https://www.sleepfoundation.org/how-sleep-works/whats-connection-between-race-and-sleep-disorders.

Suni, Eric. 2021. "Sleep Hygiene." *Sleep Foundation,* November 29. https://www.sleepfoundation.org/sleep-hygiene.

Tanner. 2021. "Journal's 'appalling' Racism Podcast, Tweet Prompt Outcry." AP NEWS, April 28. https://apnews.com/article/race-and-ethnicity-us-news-dfab22b4929d514c55a076e81ea68440.

Taylor, Keeanga-Yamahtta. 2019. *Race for Profit: How Banks and the Real Estate Industry Undermined Black Homeownership.* Chapel Hill; University of North Carolina Press.

Taylor, Lauren A., Osaze Udeagbala, Adam Biggs, Helen-Maria Lekas, and Keisha Ray. 2021. "Should a Healthcare System Facilitate Racially Concordant Care for Black Patients?" *Pediatrics 148,* no. 4 (October 1): e2021051113. https://doi.org/10.1542/peds.2021-051113.

Tessum, W. Christopher, et al. 2021. "PM 2.5 Polluters Disproportionately and Systemically Affect People of Color in the United States." *Science Advances 7* no. 18, (April 28): eabf4491. https://doi.org/10.1126/sciadv.abf4491.

The American Institute of Stress. n.d. "Stress Effects." The American Institute of Stress (blog). https://www.stress.org/stress-effects.

The Heart Foundation. 2018. "African Americans and Cardiovascular disease," September 7. https://theheartfoundation.org/2018/09/07/african-americans-and-heart-disease/.

Thomas, Jen. 2020. "Facts and Statistics on Cardiovascular disease." Healthline, July 16. https://www.healthline.com/health/heart-disease/statistics.

Tomfohr, Lianne, Meredith A. Pung, Kate M. Edwards, and Joel E. Dimsdale. 2012. "Racial Differences in Sleep Architecture: The Role of Ethnic Discrimination." *Biological Psychology 89,* no. 1 (January): 34–38. https://doi.org/10.1016/j.biopsycho.2011.09.002.

Trawalter, Sophie, Kelly M. Hoffman, and Adam Waytz. 2012. "Racial Bias in Perceptions of Others' Pain." *PLOS ONE 7,* no. 11 (November 14): 1–8. https://doi.org/10.1371/journal.pone.0048546.

Trawalter, Sophie, Kelly M. Hoffman, and Adam Waytz. 2016. "Correction: Racial Bias in Perceptions of Others' Pain." *PLOS ONE 11,* no. 3 (March 24): e0152334. https://doi.org/10.1371/journal.pone.0152334.

Traylor, Ana H., Julie A. Schmittdiel, Connie S. Uratsu, Carol M. Mangione, and Usha Subramanian. 2010. "Adherence to Cardiovascular Disease Medications: Does Patient-Provider Race/Ethnicity and Language Concordance Matter?" *Journal of General Internal Medicine 25*, no. 11 (November): 1172–77. https://doi.org/10.1007/s11606-010-1424-8.

Treede, Rolf-Detlef. 2018. "The International Association for the Study of Pain Definition of Pain: As Valid in 2018 as in 1979, but in Need of Regularly Updated Footnotes." *Pain Reports 3*, no. 2 (March 5): e643. https://doi.org/10.1097/PR9.0000000000000643.

Tweedy, Damon. 2015. *Black Man in a White Coat: A Doctor's Reflections on Race and Medicine.* New York: Picador.

U.S National Heart, Lung, and Blood Institute. 2020. "Sickle Cell Disease." September 1, 2020. https://www.nhlbi.nih.gov/health-topics/sickle-cell-disease.

U.S. Bureau of Labor Statistics. 2018. "4.9 Percent of Workers Held More than One Job at the Same Time in 2017." U.S. Department of Labor, July 19. https://www.bls.gov/opub/ted/2018/4-point-9-percent-of-workers-held-more-than-one-job-at-the-same-time-in-2017.htm.

U.S. Department of and Housing and Urban Development. 2020. *"History of Fair Housing."* U.S. Department of Housing and Urban Development (HUD). Accessed June 9. https://www.hud.gov/program_offices/fair_ho using_equal_opp/aboutfheo/history.

U.S. Department of Health and Human Services Office of Minority Health. 2021. *"Asthma and African Americans—The Office of Minority Health."* U.S. Department of Health and Human Services Office of Minority Health, November 2. https://minorityhealth.hhs.gov/omh/browse.aspx?lvl=4&lvlid=15.

U.S. Department of Health and Human Services Office of Minority Health. 2022. *"Cardiovascular disease and African Americans."* U.S. Department of Health and Human Services Office of Minority Health, January 31. https://minorityhealth.hhs.gov/omh/browse.aspx?lvl=4&lvlid=19.

United States Environmental Protection Agency. 2014. *"Children's Environmental Health Disparities: Black and African American Children and Asthma."* Overviews and Factsheets, May 20. https://www.epa.gov/child ren/childrens-environmental-health-disparities-black-and-african-ameri can-children-and-asthma.

Vera, Amir, and Laura Ly. 2020. "White Woman Who Called Police on a Black Man Bird-Watching in Central Park Has Been Fired." *CNN*, May 26. https://www.cnn.com/2020/05/26/us/central-park-video-dog-video-african-american-trnd/index.html.

Virani, Salim S., Alvaro Alonso, Emelia J. Benjamin, Marcio S. Bittencourt, Clifton W. Callaway, April P. Carson, Alanna M. Chamberlain, et al. 2020. "Cardiovascular Disease and Stroke Statistics—2020 Update: A Report

From the American Heart Association." *Circulation 141*, no. 9 (March 3). https://doi.org/10.1161/CIR.0000000000000757.

Walker, Janiece L., Roland J. Thorpe, Tracie C. Harrison, Tamara A. Baker, Michael Cary, Sarah L. Szanton, Jason C. Allaire, and Keith E. Whitfield. 2016, "The Relationship between Pain, Disability and Gender in African Americans." Clinical pain management Nursing: *Official Journal of the American Society of Clinical pain management Nurses 17*, no. 5 (October): 294–301. https://doi.org/10.1016/j.pmn.2016.05.007.

Washington, Harriet. 2006. *Medical Apartheid: The Dark History of Medical Experimentation on Black Americans from Colonial Times to the Present.* New York: First Anchor Books.

Wendland, Tegan. 2020. "New Gas and Chemical Facilities Crowd Louisiana's 'Cancer Alley.'" *NPR*, March 10, sec. Environment. https://www.npr.org/ 2020/03/10/813922168/new-gas-and-chemical-facilities-crowd-louisia nas-cancer-alley.

WHO (World Health Organization). 2012. *What are the social determinants of health?* Available at: http://www.who.int/social_determinants/sdh_definit ion/en/.

Williams, D. R. 1999. "Race, Socioeconomic Status, and Health. The Added Effects of Racism and Discrimination." *Annals of the New York Academy of Sciences 896*: 173–88. https://doi.org/10.1111/j.1749-6632.1999.tb08114.x.

Williams, David R. 1998. "African-American Health: The Role of the Social Environment." *Journal of Urban Health: Bulletin of the New York Academy of Medicine 75* (2): 300–21. https://doi.org/10.1007/BF02345099.

Williams, David R., and Toni D. Rucker. 2000. "Understanding and Addressing Racial Disparities in Health Care." *Health Care Financing Review 21* (4): 75–90.

Williams, Natasha J., Michael A. Grandne, Amy Snipes, April Rogers, Olajide Williams, Collins Airhihenbuwa, and Girardin Jean-Louis. 2015. "Racial/ Ethnic Disparities in Sleep Health and Health Care: Importance of the Sociocultural Context." *Sleep Health 1* (1): 28–35. https://doi.org/10.1016/ j.sleh.2014.12.004.

Witzig, R. 1996. "The Medicalization of Race: Scientific Legitimization of a Flawed Social Construct." *Annals of Internal Medicine 125* (8): 675–79. https://doi.org/10.7326/0003-4819-125-8-199610150-00008.

Yudell, Michael, Dorothy Roberts, Rob DeSalle, and Sarah Tishkoff. 2016. "SCIENCE AND SOCIETY. Taking Race out of Human Genetics." *Science (New York, N.Y.) 351* (6273): 564–65. https://doi.org/10.1126/science. aac4951.

Zanolli, Lauren. 2019. "'We're Just Waiting to Die': The Black Residents Living on Top of a Toxic Landfill Site." *The Guardian*, December 11, sec. US news. https://www.theguardian.com/us-news/2019/dec/11/gordon-plaza-louisi ana-toxic-landfill-site.

Zephyrin, Laurie, Shanoor Seervai, Corinne Lewis, and Jodie G. Katon. 2021. "Community-Based Models to Improve Maternal Health Outcomes and Promote Health Equity." March 4, 2021. https://doi.org/10.26099/6s6k-5330.

Zestcott, Colin A., Irene V. Blair, and Jeff Stone. 2016. "Examining the Presence, Consequences, and Reduction of Implicit Bias in Health Care: A Narrative Review." *Group Processes & Intergroup Relations: GPIR 19* (4): 528–42. https://doi.org/10.1177/1368430216642029.

Zhang, Lanlan, Elizabeth A. Reynolds Losin, Yoni K. Ashar, Leonie Koban, and Tor D. Wager. 2021. "Gender Biases in Estimation of Others' Pain." *Journal of Pain 22*, no. 9 (September): 1048–59. https://doi.org/10.1016/j.jpain.2021.03.001.

Zuberi, Tukufu. 2001. *Thicker than Blood: How Racial Statistics Lie.* Minneapolis: University of Minnesota Press.

Index

fosters ignorance amongst
clinicians, 81–82
"hardiness" narrative, 62–63
influence on next generation of
providers, 81–82
maintains clinician biases, 82
in nursing textbooks, 82
publishing ethnic stereotypes, 82
publishing false information on
race, racism, 80–81, 82
very few articles on race, racism,
81–82
medical racism, solutions for
clinician training, 78–79
education about medical racism,
78–79
listening to patients' reports, 78
medicine, 10, 64
central role in slavery, 64
denial of racism within, 79, 80
and institutional racism, 78–79
and interpersonal racism, 78–79
racism within, 5–13, 78–79, 82, 83
structural problems within, 81–82
structural racism within, 80
uncomfortable with term "racism,"
79–80
understanding of race within, 10, 11
medicine, relationship with Black
people, 6–7, 32. See also medical
racism
and historical control of
reproduction, 32
shaped by slavery, eugenics, 32
medicine, and slavery, 6–7
care of slaves, 6–7
motivated by profit, 6–7
mental health, 12, 13–14, 15, 44, 49,
117–18, 133
anxiety, 44, 45–46, 111
depression, 6–7, 44, 45–46, 53–54,
111
schizophrenia, 6–7

Michigan, 19–20
microaggressions, 19–20
migraines, 44
Mills, Charles, 138
Minneapolis (MN), 134–35
misogyny, 42
Mississippi, 19–20, 29
"Mississippi appendectomy," 29
Mitchell, Holly J., 51–52
Moffatt-Bateau, Alexandra, 67–70
Montgomery (AL), 29–30, 32–33, 34
Montgomery Community Action
Agency, 29–30
mortality, 9, 23, 88, 91–92, 109,
118–19
premature, 126
Mothers and Newborns Success Act
(2020), 52
Mothers of Gynecology (monument),
32–33
myocardial infarction, 20–21, 88–89,
108. *See also* heart attack

National Institutes of Health (NIH),
52
National Maternal Health Research
Network, 52
nausea, 107
neighborhood qualities, 19–20,
121–25. *See also* environmental
racism; environmental toxins
causing hypervigilance, 120–21,
136
crime levels, 19–20
location affects health, 130–31
noise, 120
prevent sleep, 120
shaped by racial segregation of,
124–25
New England Journal of Medicine, 81
New Orleans (Louisiana), 127–28
*New Orleans Medical and Surgical
Journal*, 62

Printed in the USA/Agawam, MA
July 17, 2023

813123.038